Rebecca Park Totilo

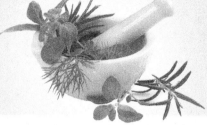

NATURE'S MEDICINE CABINET

Heal With Essential Oil

Over 125 Recipes for Treating Common Ailments Using Eight of the Most Powerful Essential Oils in Aromatherapy

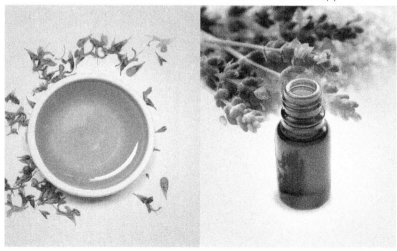

Heal With Essential Oil

Nature's Medicine Cabinet

Rebecca Park Totilo

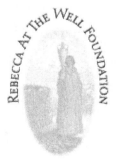

Heal With Essential Oil

Published by Rebecca at the Well Foundation
PO Box 60044
St. Petersburg, FL 33784

ISBN 978-0-9827264-0-2

Table of Contents

Nature's Medicine Cabinet

The truth regarding essential oils has long been neglected and misunderstood by most. While many Aromatherapists in the US still relegate essential oils to the support of the psyche – studies continue to confirm the tremendously powerful healing properties of essential oils for physical ailments and conditions.

Using oils drawn from nature's own medicine cabinet of flowers, trees, seeds and roots, man can tap into God's healing power to heal oneself from almost any pain, finding relief from many conditions and rejuvenate the body. Without the scientific evidence of understanding how essential oils work, we would simply call it "miraculous." Yet, simply it is since they are endowed with God's spoken word as living, vibrant substances carrying within them the healing power He offers us. As the scriptures tell us, "The Lord hath created medicines out of the earth; and he that is wise will not abhor them" (Ecclesiasticus 38:4).

Unlike over-the-counter products that fill stores' aisles, the formulas and blends you will find in this book contain no harmful chemicals. In addition, medicinal essential oils enter and leave the body with immense effectiveness and are not stored in the body like chemical drugs.

With over 125 recipes, this practical guide will walk you through in the most easy-to-understand form every conceivable use for your essential oils for everyday life. Most of the basic needs can be covered with just eight essential oils.

While essential oils are not the "magic pill" to every sickness and disease, they can work wonders for simple complaints such as colds and flu to more serious problems like arthritis and asthma.

What Are Essential Oils

Essential oils are an aromatic, vital fluid which is distilled from flowers, shrubs, leaves, trees, roots, and seeds. Because they are necessary for the life of the plant and play an important role in the biological processes of the vegetation, these substances are called "essential" and contain the essence of the plant.

The essential oil in their leaves serves two additional functions: their odors attract pollinating insects and they repel pests, bacteria, and viruses which could harm the plant. Essential oils contain the life-blood, intelligence, and vibrational energy that endow them with the healing power to sustain their own life—and help people who use them.

Unlike fatty vegetable oils used for cooking (composed of molecules too large to penetrate at a cellular level), essential oils are a non-greasy liquid composed of tiny molecules that can penetrate every cell and administer healing at the most fundamental level of our body. Their unique feature allows them to pass through the skin and cell membranes where they are most needed. Because of their structural complexity, essential oils are able to perform multiple functions just with a few drops diffused in the air or applied to the skin.

Since essential oils are derived from a natural plant source, you will notice that the oil does not leave an "oily" or greasy spot. When applied to the skin, they quickly are absorbed and go right to action. (Note: Be sure to check safety ratings before applying any essential oil to the skin.)

Modern medicine has attempted to duplicate the chemical constituents and healing capabilities of essential oils, but cannot. Man-made pharmaceuticals lack the intelligence and life-force found in the healing oils. Most synthetic prescriptions have multiple undesirable side effects—even some that are deadly.

Essential oils have no serious side effects that are deadly. Many people have reported authentic healing when using them—though everyone may not experience the same results as family history, lifestyle, and diet plays a significant role in the body's healing process. Essential oils work together in harmony, making them inherently safe, unlike when multiple prescription drugs are taken, causing drug-interaction, other health issues and sometimes even death.

Essential Oil Safety

In general, essential oils are safe to use for aromatherapy and other household purposes. Nonetheless, safety must be exercised due to their potency and high concentration. Please read and follow these guidelines to receive the maximum effectiveness and benefits.

- Avoid applying essential oils immediately after perspiring or using a sauna.

- Remember the Sabbath. Take a break from using essentials oil once a week. Use them six days, and then take one day off.

- Be careful to not get essential oils in the eyes. If you do splash a drop or two of essential oil in the eyes, use a small amount of olive oil (or another carrier oil) to dilute the essential oil and absorb with a wash cloth. If serious, seek medical attention immediately.

- Always keep your essential oils out of reach from children. Take special precaution when using oils with children. Never use undiluted essential oils on babies.

- If a dangerous quantity of essential oil is ingested, immediately drink olive oil and induce vomiting. The olive oil will help in slowing down its absorption and dilute the essential oil. Do not drink water—this will speed up the absorption of the essential oil.

- Take extra precaution when using essential oils during pregnancy or if suffering from a terminal illness.

- The nose knows—if you don't like a fragrance, then don't use it for emotional benefits.

• Some essential oils should be diluted before applying topically. Pay attention to safety guidelines—certain essential oils, such as Cinnamon and Clove, may cause skin irritation for those with sensitive skin. If you experience slight redness or itchiness, put olive oil (or any carrier oil) on the affected area and cover with a soft cloth. The olive oil acts as an absorbent fat and binds to the oil, diluting its effect and allowing it to be quickly removed. Aloe Vera gel also works well as an alternative to olive oil. Never use water to dilute essential oil—this will cause it to spread and enlarge the affected area. Redness or irritation may last 20 minutes to an hour.

• It is recommended to only apply certain essential oils directly to the skin undiluted in certain circumstances and in specific conditions. Please exercise caution and apply only properly diluted essential oils to the skin, and follow the recipes and methods carefully.

• Keep oils away from heat, light, moisture and elec-tromagnetic fields (television, microwave, etc.).

• For sensitive skin, do a "patch test." If irritation oc-curs, discontinue use of such oil or blend.

• Avoid sunbathing or tanning booths immediately af-ter using essential oils.

• Use essential oils that match your largest number of needs.

• Never take essential oils internally, unless advised by your medical practitioner or another qualified health profes-sional.

• If you are pregnant, lactating, suffer from epilepsy or high blood pressure, have cancer, liver damage, or another medical condition, use essential oils under the care and supervision of a qualified aroma-therapist or medical practitioner. Some oils may have a stimulating effect on the urinary system and uterus, since essential oils are able to cross the placental barrier. In addition, while nursing a baby, be careful to prevent skin transference to baby and/or through the mother's milk.

• Be sure to not get essential oils on any mucous membranes. Wash hands after handling pure, undiluted essential oils.

• If taking prescription drugs, check for interaction between medicine and essential oils (if any) to avoid interference with certain prescription medications.

• To avoid contact sensitization (redness or irritation of skin due to repeated use of same individual oil) rotate and use different oils.

• Keep essential oil vials and clear glass bottles in a box or another dark place for storing.

• For high hypertension (high blood pressure) and diabetic patients, please check safety ratings of essentials oils before use.

Safety Guidelines

       Essential oils are distilled from plant leaves, flowers, roots, seeds, bark and resins, or are expressed from the rinds of citrus fruits. It generally takes at least 50 pounds of plant material to make one pound of essential oil (for example, a pound of Rosemary oil requires sixty-six pounds of herb), but the ratio is sometimes astonishing - it takes 2,300 pounds of rose flowers petals to make a single pound of oil.

       Because they contain no fatty acids, essential oils are not susceptible to rancidity like vegetable oils - but protect them from the degenerative effects of heat, light and air; store them in tightly sealed, dark glass bottles away from any heat source. Properly stored oils can maintain their quality for years. (Citrus oils are less stable and should not be stored longer than six months after opening.)

ESSENTIAL OIL TIPS

1. Always read and follow all label warnings and cautions.

2. Keep oils tightly closed and out of the reach of children.

3. Never consume undiluted oils. Cook only with essential oils approved as a food additive and considered generally regarded as safe (GRAS).

4. Don't use undiluted oils on your skin. (Dilute with carrier oil).

5. Skin test oils before using. Dilute a small amount and apply to the skin on your inner arm. Do not use if redness or irritation occurs.

6. Keep oils away from eyes and mucous membranes.

7. If redness, burning, itching, or irritation occurs, stop using oil immediately.

8. Avoid use of these oils during pregnancy: Bitter Almond, Basil, Clary Sage, Clove Bud, Hyssop, Sweet Fennel, Juniper Berry, Marjoram, Myrrh, Peppermint, Rose, Rosemary, Sage, Thyme and Wintergreen.

9. These oils can be especially irritating to the skin: Allspice, Bitter Almond, Basil, Cinnamon Leaf, Cinnamon Bark, Clove Bud, Sweet Fennel, Fir needle, Lemon, Lemongrass, Melissa, Peppermint, Tea Tree and Wintergreen. In addition, Angelica and all citrus oils make the skin more sensitive to ultraviolet light. Do not go out into the sun with these oils on your skin.

10. Sweet Fennel, Hyssop, Rosemary and Sage essential oils should not be used by anyone with epilepsy. People with high blood pressure should avoid Hyssop, Rosemary, Sage and Thyme essential oils.

11. For someone who tends to be highly allergic, here is a simple test to use to help determine if he/she is sensitive to particular oil. First, rub a drop of carrier oil onto the upper chest. In 12 hours, check for redness or other skin irritation. If the skin remains clear, place 1 drop of selected essential oil in 15 drops of the same carrier oil, and again rub into the upper chest. If no skin reaction appears after 12 hours, it's probably safe to use the carriers and the essential oil.

12. After applying citrus oils to the skin, avoid exposure to sunlight, since the oils may burn the skin.

13. When spilled on furniture, many essential oils will remove the finish. It's best to be careful when handling the bottles.

14. Don't buy perfume oils thinking they are the same thing as essential oils. Perfume oils do not offer the therapeutic benefits of essential oils. Even if you only intend on using aromatherapy in your lifestyle for the sheer enjoyment of the aroma, essential oils that are breathed in can offer therapeutic benefits. These benefits do not occur with the use of perfume oils.

15. Don't buy essential oils with rubber glass dropper tops. Essential oils are very concentrated and will turn the rubber to a gum thus ruining the oil.

16. It is also helpful to note the country of origin for the oil. Most good essential oil sellers will readily supply the botanical names and country of origin for the oils that they sell. When comparing one company's oils with another's, also pay attention to if either company's oils are organic, wild-crafted or ethically farmed.

17. It is wise not to purchase oils from vendors at street fairs, craft shows, or other limited-time events. Some vendors know beginners have no recourse against them later. This is not to say that there are not highly reputable sellers at such events, but this is a caution for beginners who are not able to reliably judge quality.

18. Be selective of where you purchase your essential oils. The quality of essential oils varies widely from company to company. Additionally, some companies may falsely claim that their oils are undiluted or pure when they aren't. We recommend you purchase your essential oils from http://HealWithOil.com.

19. If essential oil is ingested, rinse mouth out with milk, and then drink a large glass of milk. Seek medical advice immediately. If essential oil gets into eyes, flush with large quantity of water immediately. Seek medical advice immediately. If

essential oils are splashed onto skin and irritation results, apply carrier oil to the area to dilute.

Safety Ratings

We use only essential oils that have been obtained from a highly-reputable company that have a safety code to identify additional safety precautions for each essential oil.

A: Generally considered safe.

B: Skin irritant (strong) and mucous membranes irritant (moderate). Restrict level of use in products.

C: Skin and mucous membrane irritant. Dilution required.

D: Oil may cause skin irritation in people with very sensitive skin or damaged skin, or can cause an allergic reaction.

E: Very sensitizing allergen which could cause dermatitis. Use caution.

F: Oil should be used in moderation due to toxicity levels.

G: Photosensitivity—direct exposure to sunlight after use could cause dermatitis.

H: Hazardous oral toxin.

I: Avoid if you have high blood pressure.

J: Avoid if you have epilepsy.

K: No formal testing. Use caution.

L: Avoid if you have diabetes.

Dilution Rate Chart

This dilution rate chart shows you the percentage of pure therapeutic essential oil to use to the number of drops of carrier oil (vegetable oil) and will help you convert essential and carrier oil measurements. Use a measuring cup or spoon for carrier oils and pipettes for measuring your essential oils.

It is important to dilute your essential oil for mixing with a suitable carrier oil, so that you can use it on the skin over a part of the body. There are different carrier oils (such as Sweet Almond, Cold Pressed Extra Virgin Olive, Flaxseed, Avocado, Grapeseed Extract, Jojoba, etc.) and you will want to select the best one for your purpose and skin type. Carrier oils can be purchased from a natural health food store or grocer, but check labels to make sure the one you select is cold pressed oil and is suitable for use on the skin.

For general purposes, the dilution rate for essential oils is generally 2% - 3%. For instance, if you use two-three drops of pure essential oil, you will dilute by adding about a teaspoon of carrier oil. This should be cut in half for children and senior citizens.

Simple Everyday Dilution Chart:

2-3 drops of Essential Oil per teaspoon of Carrier Oil
7-8 drops of Essential Oil per Tablespoon of Carrier Oil
15 drops of Essential Oil per Ounce (30ml) of Carrier Oil

Two to three drops of essential oils is the most you should use in an eight-hour period. Keep in mind, less is best when it comes to essential oils, and it would be wasteful to use more.

5% Dilution Rate (approximate)

1 ounce carrier oil (2 Tablespoons) + 1.5 ml essential oil
2 ounce carrier oil (1/4 cup) + 3 ml essential oil
3 ounce carrier oil (1/3 cup) + 4.5 ml essential oil
4 ounce carrier oil (1/2 cup) + 6 ml essential oil
8 ounce carrier oil (1 cup) + 9 ml essential oil

10% Dilution Rate (approximate)

1 ounce carrier oil (2 Tablespoons) + 3 ml essential oil
2 ounce carrier oil (1/4 cup) + 6 ml essential oil
3 ounce carrier oil (1/3 cup) + 9 ml essential oil
4 ounce carrier oil (1/2 cup) + 12 ml essential oil
8 ounce carrier oil (1 cup) + 24 ml essential oil

ML Conversion to Ounces (approximate drops)

1 ml = 20-24 drops
3 ml = .10 ounce (approximately 60-72 drops)
6 ml = .20 ounce (approximately 120-144 drops)
9 ml = .30 ounce (approximately 180-216 drops)
12 ml = .40 ounce (approximately 240-288 drops)
24 ml = .80 ounce (approximately 480-576 drops)

Teaspoons to Drops

1/8 teaspoon = 12.5 drops = 1/48 ounce = 5/8 ml
1/4 teaspoon = 25 drops = 1/24 ounce = 1 1/4 ml
3/4 teaspoon = 75 drops = 1/8 ounce = 3.7 ml
1 teaspoon = 100 drops = 1/6 ounce = 5 ml

Quick Conversions

3 teaspoons (tsp) = 1 Tablespoon (tbsp)
2 tablespoons (tbsp) = 1 ounce (oz)
6 teaspoons (tsp) = 1 ounce (oz)
10 milliliter (ml) = 1/3 ounce (oz)
15 milliliter (ml) = 1/2 ounce (oz)
30 milliliter (ml) = 1 ounce (oz)
10 milliliter (ml) = approximately 300 drops

Pregnant Women

For women who are pregnant, the general rule is a one percent (1%) dilution for oils that are safe to use. For a 3.5 ounce bottle (100 ml) carrier oil, add 25 drops essential oil and for 1/3 ounce carrier oil (10 ml or 2 teaspoons), add 2 drops essential oil.

Massage Oil

When you use essential oils for a massage, you will need to dilute with a carrier oil. Generally, two drops of essential oil (use only Therapeutic Grade Essential Oils) should be used per teaspoon of Carrier Oil (but follow individual recipes if available). A full body massage takes about one to two ounces of carrier oil. Any natural carrier oil (except mineral oil) is fine to use when preparing a massage blend. As a general rule, add 10-12 drops of essential oil to 30ml of carrier oil. For children and elderly, use only 5-7 drops of essential oil to 30ml of carrier oil.

Blending Oils For Therapeutic Use

Creating your own fragrance or blend using your essential oils will be one of your most satisfying aspects in using your oils.

There are two types of blending you can do: therapeutic and aromatic. Whether you are blending for therapeutic benefits or just for aroma, be sure to pay close attention to the contraindications of any essential oil you choose and safety guidelines regarding its use. For instance, if you are creating a blend to aid in an upper respiratory condition (such as congestion) but suffer from epilepsy, you will not want to use Rosemary as it could cause a seizure.

You will also want to make sure the essential oils you choose for your blend won't contradict the effect you desire. For instance, if you are creating a blend to enhance deep sleep, you want to avoid using oils that spark energy (such as Lemon), keeping you alert and awake.

The aromatic description listed under each essential oil, along with its use, will help you get started. For more information, there are several books available online and at your local bookstore that can provide you with greater detail and information on how to use and blend oils. It will be worth the investment to get several resources and have them on hand for the days ahead.

Creating a blend of essential oils for therapeutic properties will aid you with physical and emotional conditions. Your focus will be more on the healing benefits of the oil rather than its aroma—although the aroma of your blend will bring more desirable results when it is something you enjoy using.

Follow these simple steps to help you get started:

1. Pray and ask the Father for His guidance and direction as you create your formula. This blend will be uniquely yours and He will use these oils to reach into the deepest areas of your body, soul, and spirit.

2. Have a notebook and pencil handy to write down the formula. (Trust me, you will forget how many drops you used of each oil if you don't do this.) Write down how many drops of each fragrance you use, so you will know the final formula of your blend and can duplicate it later. Give your fragrance a name.

3. Using an empty, clean bottle, start small—use only 5 to 10 drops. This way, if you end up not liking the blend you have created, you won't have wasted too much.

4. Don't add your carrier oil until you have finished blending your essential oils. Once you have designed your blend, you can add your favorite carrier oil. This way you don't waste the carrier oil if you end up not liking the aroma you created. Shake well to mix and let set for a day or two to breathe.

5. Add a label to your bottle with your fragrance name.

Quick Reference Blending Chart

Here's a quick guide to how much essential oil to use for each application. For recipes and formulas, be sure to follow amounts listed in the directions. Caution: For children, elderly and pregnant women, please divide essential oil amount in half for body applications.

Method	Carrier/Amount	Essential Oils Drops
Vaporizer	Full	5 to 10
Humidifier	Full	5 to 10
Steam Inhalation	Full Bowl	2 to 3
Diffuser/Nebulizer	-	10 to 25
Stove Top	Full Pan	6 to 12
Light Ring	-	1 to 2
Tea Lights/Burner	-	4 to 6
Vacuum Cleaner	Bag/Filter	3 to 5
Room Spray	4 Ounces	80 to 100
Household Cleaner	8 Ounces	80 to 100
Body Lotion	4 Ounces	25
Body Oil	4 Ounces	50
Massage Oil	1 Tablespoon	7 to 10
Shampoo	1 Ounces	10
Conditioner	1 Ounce	10
Chest Rub	1 Ounces	15 to 25
Compress	-	8 to 10
Tissue	-	1 to 2
Mouthwash	1 Teaspoon	2 to 3
Foot Bath/Spa	Small Tub	5
Bath	Full Tub	8 to 10
Shower	Washcloth	1 to 2
Sauna	1 Cup Water	1 to 2
Hot Tub/Jacuzzi	Full	10 to 15

Methods of Use

Direct Inhalation
Apply 2-3 drops of essential oils into your hand and rub palms together. Cup hands over nose and mouth. Inhale vapors deeply several times.

Humidifier/Vaporizer
For a humidifier or vaporizer, place 10 drops of essential oil undiluted into the unit.

Hot Tubs/Jacuzzi
Add 10 drops of your favorite essential oil to your hot tub or Jacuzzi.

Linens/Blankets
Add your favorite essential oil to a spray bottle with water and spray to freshen bed sheets and blankets at bedtime and enhance deep sleep.

Household Cleaners
Use essential oils as disinfectants for natural, non-chemical cleaners. This will kill airborne virus and strengthen the immune system, and deodorize the area with wonderful eco-friendly fragrances.

Light Bulb Rings
When using a metal light bulb ring, use six drops of essential oil and just enough water to prevent burning. Add a little water first, then drop the essential oil on top to float on water. If you are using a porcelain light ring, you may not

need to add any water. Take into consideration the size or wattage of the bulb, as some will get warmer. Place ring over light bulb when light is cool and be sure to not get essential oil directly on light bulb.

Pottery/Electric Burners

A wide variety of burners are available to use—some electric, some using tea light candles. Generally, tea light candles are not too hot for diffusing essential oils, but you may want to drop oils over glass stones or add water to the top section to help diffuse fragrance. Use caution around open fire, as essential oils are flammable. Six drops of oils is recommended for normal use; however, you may want to reduce the amount of oil used for rooms of elderly or children.

Nebulizing Diffuser/Cool Mist

Place 25 drops of essential oil undiluted inside and use as needed. Limit diffusion of new oils to 10 minutes each day, increasing the time until desired effects are reached. Adjust times for different-sized rooms and the strength of each fragrance. Unlike the cheap fragrant oils purchased at department stores that mask odors, diffusing pure essential oils actually alters the structure of the molecules that create odors – rendering them harmless. Essential oils increase the available oxygen in the room and produce negative ions which kill microbes. Do not use thick essential oils in your diffuser, as this could possibly clog it.

Sitz Bath/Bath

To help treat problems in the pelvic or genital areas, try adding 5 drops of essential oil in just enough water to cover lower body. For a full bath, add 8-10 drops of essential oil while bath is running. Agitate water in a figure eight motion to make sure the oil is mixed well, preventing irritation to mucous membranes. Another method is to add essential oils after the bath has been drawn. Add essential oils with a palm full of liquid soap or shampoo and swishing around to dissolve in tub. Soak for 15-20 minutes.

Shower
While showering, add a drop or two of essential oil to a washcloth and rub on body.

Compress
Dilute 1 part essential oil with 4 parts carrier oil (olive oil works great) and apply 8-10 drops on affected area. Using a moist towel or washcloth, cover with a dry towel and leave on for 10 minutes. For inflammation, use a cold compress. If there is no inflammation, use a warm compress.

Facial Steam/Steam Inhalation
Place 2-3 drops of essential oil in a bowl of hot water. Place towel over your head and inhale for 5 minutes. Be careful to use only safe oils, as some essential oils may irritate the eyes. This type of treatment is also beneficial if you are suffering from a cold or upper respiration ailment.

Lotions /Creams
Blending essential oils in an unscented, natural lotion/cream base allows you to benefit from the therapeutic qualities of the essential oil, giving you a non-oily way to apply essential oils. This is particularly beneficial for someone with a skin condition that doesn't do well with oils. The dilution rate for using essential oils in a lotion base is no more than 2%. For adults, use 20 drops of essential oil to 50g of lotion. For

children and elderly, use 10 drops of essential oil to 50g of lotion.

Massage Stones

Here's an inexpensive spa treatment you can do at home. Select a flat smooth stone the size of your palm, and heat in the oven at a low temperature until warm. Rub a massage oil blend (10-15 drops of essential oil per one-ounce of carrier oil) over the heated rock to give your spouse a relaxing massage to penetrate muscles (Himalayan Salt Stones work great for this).

Body Oils

Mix 30 drops of essential oil per one ounce of cold-pressed carrier oil such as olive oil. Choose an all-purpose oil that is great for the muscles, relieves pain, headache, and tension and smells lovely.

Sprays/Spritzers

Creating your own body sprays and facial mists is one of the easiest ways to use essential oils. For a facial mist, use 8-10 drops of essential oils in a four-ounce spray bottle filled with distilled water. For body sprays, add 30-40 drops of essential oil per four-ounce spray bottle filled with distilled water. For room sprays, use 80-100 drops of essential oil per four-ounce spray bottle with the remainder filled with distilled water. Be careful not to spray in the eyes.

Stovetop

Fill a saucepan with ¾ with water and add six drops of oil to pan. Set stove setting on "warm." Check periodically to make sure water has not evaporated.

Gargle/Mouthwash

Add 3 drops of essential oil to 1 teaspoon of water to use as a mouthwash.

Massage

A variety of techniques used in massage therapy can incorporate the use of essential oils. Refer to the list of therapeutic properties for which oils you will find most beneficial and add 7 drops of essential oil to 1 tablespoon to massage oil.

Remedies Chart

Acne: Tea Tree, Lavender, Eucalyptus and Clove

Allergies: Lavender, Rosemary

Anxiety: Lavender, Eucalyptus

Arthritis: Eucalyptus, Lavender, Lemon and Rosemary

Artistic Condition: Clove, Cinnamon and Peppermint

Asthma: Eucalyptus, Lavender, Peppermint and Tea Tree

Back Pain: Clove, Lavender, Peppermint and Rosemary

Bruises: Clove, Lavender

Burns: Clove, Eucalyptus, Tea Tree and Lavender

Candida: Eucalyptus, Tea Tree and Lavender, Cinnamon, Clove, Peppermint and Rosemary

Cellulite: Lemon, Eucalyptus, Peppermint, Rosemary

Colds and Flu: Lemon, Peppermint, Clove, Tea Tree, Rosemary, Eucalyptus and Lavender

Cold Sores: Tea Tree, Clove and Cinnamon

Cuts: Clove, Eucalyptus, Lavender and Lemon

Dandruff Treatment: Rosemary, Tea Tree and Lavender

Depression: Lavender, Cinnamon and Peppermint

Dermatitis: Lavender, Peppermint

Detoxify: Peppermint, Rosemary and Lemon

Diabetes: Cinnamon, Rosemary, Lavender (used with Doc In the Box Blend)

Eczema: Tea Tree, Lavender

Emotional Discomfort: Cinnamon, Lemon and Rosemary

Epidermophytia: Clove, Eucalyptus, Lavender and Lemon

Epstein-Barr Syndrome or Virus: Cinnamon, Clove, Lemon, Tea Tree, Rosemary and Lavender

Eye Strain/Exhaustion: Cinnamon, Lemon, Rosemary

Fatigue: Lavender, Lemon, Eucalyptus, Peppermint and Rosemary

Fever: Lemon, Lavender, Eucalyptus, Tea Tree, Rosemary and Peppermint

Grief: Rosemary

Gloomy Feeling: Lavender

Hair Loss: Lavender, Rosemary and Eucalyptus

Headaches: Eucalyptus, Lavender, Rosemary, Lemon and Peppermint

Heart Attack: Lavender, Peppermint and Lemon

Herpes: Eucalyptus, Lemon and Tea Tree

High Blood Pressure: Lavender, Lemon and Cinnamon

Immune Deficiency: Lavender, Lemon, Rosemary, Tea Tree and Eucalyptus

Inability to Concentrate: Rosemary, Peppermint, Lemon

Indecision: Eucalyptus, Rosemary

Infection (Bacterial or Viral): Tea Tree (with Rosemary), Lemon, Lavender, Eucalyptus, Clove, Cinnamon and Doc In A Box Blend

Insect Bites: Tea Tree, Lavender and Eucalyptus

Insomnia: Lavender

Irritability: Lavender

Lice: Eucalyptus (with Lavender or Peppermint)

Malaria: Lemon

Melanoma: Lavender

Memory: Rosemary, Peppermint and Lemon

Menstrual Cramps: Lavender, Rosemary, Peppermint

Motion Sickness: Lavender, Peppermint and Rosemary

Nausea: Cinnamon, Clove, Lavender and Peppermint

Nervous Exhaustion: Peppermint, Rosemary (better to inhale from the vial)

Oily Hair: Rosemary, Lemon

Open Pores: Lemon, Peppermint

Overindulgence: Lemon, Peppermint, Tea Tree and Eucalyptus

Pest Control/Insects: Clove, Lavender and Lemon

Physical Exhaustion: Rosemary (bath, massage)

Pigmentation: Lemon, Tea Tree

Pneumonia: Lavender (with Lemon or Peppermint), Tea Tree (with Cinnamon)

Polio: Lemon

Poison Ivy/Oak: Peppermint, Eucalyptus, Tea Tree and Rosemary

Psoriasis: Lavender, Clove, Tea Tree and Rosemary

Rashes: Lavender, Tea Tree

Recall and Memory: Rosemary, Peppermint, Clove and Lemon

Shingles: Clove, Thyme, Peppermint, Eucalyptus and Lavender

Scabies: Lavender, Peppermint and Rosemary

Shock: Peppermint, Tea Tree (with Lavender)

Scars and Stretch Marks: Lavender

Skin (flabby/fatty): Rosemary, Lemon

Skin (irritated): Lavender, Tea Tree

Sprains: Lemon and Peppermint

Strep: Cinnamon (with Lavender), Doc In The Box Blend

Stress: Lavender, Rosemary

Teeth Whitening: Lemon

Tropical Infections: Cinnamon, Tea Tree

Typhoid: Cinnamon, Peppermint

Uplifting: Rosemary

Warts and Calluses: Lavender, Lemon and Tea Tree

Weakness: Rosemary

Weight Loss: Lemon, Rosemary

Wounds: Clove, Eucalyptus, Lavender, Rosemary, Peppermint, Tea Tree and Doc In The Box Blend

Cinnamon Essential Oil

Cinnamomum zeylanicum, Cinnamon's botanical name, comes from trees native to China and South East Asia. Its use is recorded in Chinese journals as early as 2700 B.C. During the middle ages, the Arabs that traded Cinnamon preserved their monopoly of the spice trade by claiming it was harvested from the nest of ferocious birds while under attack. Many believe Cinnamon attracts wealth and prosperity.

Obtained from its bark or leaf, the reddish brown spicy oil warms the heart with its ability to help the melancholia and lift one's spirit from depression caused by lethargy and lack of vitality. Cinnamon is revered for its antiseptic properties and is best known for the treatment of stomach ailments including a sluggish digestive system, flatulence and intestinal disorders.

Medical research reveals Cinnamon can lower blood glucose and help with the metabolism in controlling diabetes. Some recent studies have shown that if you consume as little as ½ teaspoon of Cinnamon powder each day you may be able to reduce blood sugar, cholesterol and triglyceride levels by as much as 20%. Some believe it is a substance known as MHCP that causes Cinnamon to reignite the body's fat cells to respond to insulin and this dramatically increases the removal of glucose. Other studies being conducted reveal new evidence that it acts as an anti-inflammatory agent, along with being an anti-oxidant agent, which can lower cholesterol, triglycerides and glucose as well as improve the functioning of insulin in the body. (Please note: Cinnamon essential is 70-80 times more potent than Cinnamon powder, see application for dilution rate.)

While Cinnamon is used more extensively in cooking and flavoring of beverages because of its pleasant taste than in aromatherapy, it certainly has its place for combating viral and infectious diseases.

In the book, Cinnamon and Cassia, by P. N. Ravindran, K. Nirmal Babu, M. Shylaja the authors stated:

"The different investigations reveal that Cinnamon shows both immune system potentiating and inhibiting effects. Kaishi-ni-eppi-ichi tu, a Chinese herbal preparation containing Cinnamon as its main constituent, has been shown to exhibit antiviral action against the influenza A2 virus."

According to "The Journal of Agricultural and Food Chemistry," Cinnamon essential oil makes an excellent mosquito repellent because of its high concentration of cinnamaldehyde, an active mosquito killing agent.

Cinnamon blends well with Frankincense, Orange, Lemon, Rosemary, Lavender and Onycha (Benzoin).

Plant Origin: China, Southeast Asia, India

Medicinal Properties: Anti-microbial, anti-infectious, antibacterial (for large spectrum of infection), antiseptic, anti-inflammatory, antiviral, antifungal, anticoagulant, antidepressant, and emotional stimulant.

Traditional Uses: Fungal infections (Candida), general tonic, and increases blood flow when previously restricted. Good for digestive system, calms spasms, high blood pressure, colitis, flatulence, diarrhea and nausea. It is known to ease muscular spasms and painful rheumatic joints, as well as general aches and pains. It also affects the libido and is known as an aphrodisiac. Several studies suggest that Cinnamon may have a regulatory effect on blood sugar, making it especially beneficial for people with type II diabetes. In some studies, Cinnamon has shown an amazing ability to stop medication-resistant yeast infections. In a study published by researchers at the U.S. Department of Agriculture in Maryland, Cinnamon reduced the proliferation of leukemia and lymphoma cancer cells. It has shown to have an anti-clotting effect on the blood.

Application: Dilute 1 part essential oil with 4 parts carrier oil and apply one to two drops on location; diffuse; or massage. Cinnamon may be used in food or beverage as a dietary supplement. Capsule, 0 size.

Caution: This oil may be a potent skin irritant (skin may turn red or burn)—be sure to dilute with carrier oil. Because of its high phenol content, it is best diluted (1 drop to 40 or 50 drops of a carrier oil, such as extra-virgin olive oil) before applying to the skin. If the mixture is too hot, apply additional diluting oil. Use extreme care as it may irritate the nasal membranes if inhaled directly from diffuser or bottle. Avoid during pregnancy.

Safety Rating: C

Uses for Cinnamon Essential Oil

1. Rub a drop or two of Cinnamon essential oil mixed in carrier oil to calm spasms of the digestive tract, indigestion, or nausea.

2. Add a drop of Cinnamon essential oil to a dried flower arrangement or potpourri to spice up the home. Researchers found that just having the scent in a room helps to reduces drowsiness, irritability, and the pain and frequency of headaches.

3. Cinnamon essential oil can be used in cooking. It also increases the action of enzymes that break down food in the body, aiding in the metabolic process.

4. Place a drop or two of Cinnamon essential oil in a light bulb ring for help with mental clarity and concentration.

5. When your body feels achy, add one drop of Cinnamon essential oil to 4 parts carrier oil to provide heat, relax tight muscles, ease painful joints, and relieve menstrual cramps.

6. To help fight viral, fungal, and bacterial illnesses and to boost the immune system, diffuse in the kitchen. Wipe kitchen sinks down with Cinnamon essential oil to kill virus or bacteria growth.

7. Blend Cinnamon essential oil with other fragrances such as Lavender, Frankincense, or another favorite with olive oil and apply to a handkerchief to carry with you and inhale as necessary on airplane flights.

8. Use Cinnamon essential oil for head lice. For preventive treatment, add 4 drops to a mixture of 1 ounce vinegar and 1 ounce of water. Use as a hair rinse. (Be sure to not get

Cinnamon essential oil in the eyes or burn your scalp. Perform a skin patch test, especially on children to prevent skin irritation.)

9. Diffuse Cinnamon essential oil in the home or office to lift spirits. Cinnamon essential oil is known to be a natural antidepressant.

10. To treat fungal infections such as athlete's foot, use a drop or two of Cinnamon essential oil on the feet or add essential oil to a foot bath.

11. As a general immunity stimulant, add a few drops of Cinnamon essential oil to a pan of water and simmer to fill your home with its warm aroma.

12. Stay on track by filling your exercise room or gym with Cinnamon essential oil to increase stamina.

13. When using Cinnamon essential oil in massage oil, dilute at 1% to prevent burning or irritating skin. This will help strengthen your immune system.

14. Simmer a couple of drops of Cinnamon essential oil on the stovetop to ward off colds, flu, and other airborne infections and contagious diseases.

15. To alleviate melancholia, lethargy, or lack of energy, use Cinnamon essential oil in a diffuser.

16. Add a drop of Cinnamon essential oil to your tea on a regular basis to help your blood glucose come down and control diabetes. Add ginger for the prevention of a cold or flu.

17. Got Candida? Try Cinnamon or Cassia essential oil. Studies show how Cinnamon help stops the growth of

bacteria as well as fungi, including the commonly problematic yeast Candida which many women suffer from.

18. Cinnamon is proven to boost brain activity. Just sniff and experience the difference in your cognitive processing.

19. An effective way to relieve digestive problems is to use Cinnamon essential oil in an abdominal massage oil. It stimulates the circulation, especially to the extremities and promotes a general sense of vitality.

20. Cinnamon makes a wonderful room fragrance. Add 8-10 drops of Cinnamon essential oil to a spray bottle with distilled water. The strong antiseptic properties of Cinnamon make it a valuable room fumigant protection against flu viruses.

21. Soothe sore muscles with a massage using two table-spoons of Grapeseed oil and a couple drops of Cinnamon essential oil. Massage briskly to stimulate circulation and flush away toxins.

22. Diffuse Cinnamon essential oil in a burner or vaporizer for acute bronchitis and colds.

23. Trouble concentrating? Diffuse two drops of Cinnamon, two drops of Rosemary and five drops of Lemon essential oil in an electric burner.

24. Got cold hands and feet at night? Place a drop of Cinnamon essential oil on the tongue or take a pinch of Cinnamon powder.

25. To repel flies, apply diluted Cinnamon essential oil to exposed skin and dab on clothing.

Peppermint Essential Oil

Known for its minty fresh leaves, *Mentha piperita* better know as Peppermint is used in a wide variety of applications, including teas and other beverages, soaps, shampoos, cigarettes, toothpastes, ice creams, candies, medicines, cosmetics, and chewing gums. Its effect on the digestive system is one of the reasons for its popularity as a favorite ingredient in after-dinner mints and chewing gums. Peppermint is refreshing, stimulating, and promotes clarity and alertness.

Studies at the University of Cincinnati revealed Peppermint essential oil improved concentration and mental alertness. Alan Hirsch, MD also discovered this oil helps to trigger the brain's satiety center in hypothalamus which gives the body a sense of fullness after a meal.

Because of its mostly cool menthol content (85%), Peppermint is found in most liniments to relieve painful muscle spasms and arthritic conditions. Its energetic scent was said to be an aphrodisiac in ancient times.

In Egypt, Peppermint was found in tombs dating from 1000 BCE. As one of the oldest herbs used for digestion, Peppermint is extremely effective against stomach ailments and helps with gaseous indigestion and an irritated colon. Its antispasmodic action relieves the smooth muscles of the stomach and gut, aiding with stomach pain, vomiting, and diarrhea. It is also successful in treatment for odorous gas due to intestinal parasites or Candida. Peppermint essential oil is also great for headaches, fevers, colds and flu. In addition, this pale white oil is hepatic and works to detoxify the liver.

Peppermint essential oil contains numerous minerals and nutrients including manganese, calcium, iron, magnesium, folate, potassium, and copper. It also contains omega-3 fatty acids, Vitamin A and Vitamin C.

Peppermint essential oil blends well with Lavender, Rosemary, Eucalyptus, and Lemon essential oils.

Plant Origin: America, Germany, France, Japan

Medicinal Properties: Analgesic, antibacterial, antifungal, anti-inflammatory, anti-infectious, antiphlogistic, antiseptic, antispasmodic, antidepressant, astringent, carminative, decongestant, expectorant, febrifuge, nervine, stomachic, digestive, stimulants the gallbladder and vasoconstrictor.

Traditional Uses: Research was conducted by Jean Valnet, M.D. on Peppermint's effect on the liver and respiratory system as one of the most valued herbs. Ongoing research at the University of Cincinnati and other universities on Peppermint's role in affecting impaired taste and smell when inhaled and its ability to improve concentration and mental accuracy continues.

Other Uses: Aids in concentration, acts as a stimulant, beneficial in digestive issues such as irritable bowel syndrome, nausea, diarrhea, food poisoning and motion sickness. Peppermint is also great for headaches, fevers, throat infections, bronchitis, colds and flu. Peppermint works well to relieve muscle, arthritic and menstrual pain and irregularity because of the cooling effect constricting the capillaries. It also improves blood circulation. Other uses include: Candida, palpitations, asthma, dizziness, fainting, flatulence, indigestion, ringworm, toothaches, bad breath, laryngitis, heartburn, hemorrhoids, hot flashes, headaches, hypotension, hysteria, kidney and gallstones. It helps with morning sickness and decreases lactation in nursing mothers. Peppermint essential oil stimulates oil production in dry skin and hair. Many bacterial, viral and fungal infections are destroyed by inhaling Peppermint or when rubbed on the chest in a balm. It supports the immune system.

Application: Apply topically, take orally, massaged, in a bath or diffuse. Take orally for indigestion, abdominal cramping, gas, acid reflux, intestinal parasites, or bad breath.

Safety: Can possibly be a skin irritant if too much is applied. Be sure to dilute. Avoid if pregnant or nursing a baby.

Safety Rating: D

Uses For Peppermint Essential Oil

1. Place one drop of Peppermint Essential Oil on your tongue for bad breath or after a meal to freshen breath.

2. Peppermint relieves diarrhea or other digestive ailments, including indigestion. Place one or two drops on tummy or on tongue for instant relief. Inhaling Peppermint is also great for nausea.

3. To relieve aches all over the body, blend several drops of Peppermint essential oil with a carrier oil and massage into muscles.

4. Peppermint works wonders for headaches. Inhale deeply from an open bottle or place one or two drops of Peppermint essential oil on the temples or back of the neck.

5. Peppermint is great for recovering from jet lag. It resets your body's clock and helps you recover quicker for a long trip.

6. Always carry Peppermint essential oil with you while traveling in a car to help prevent motion sickness. Massage several drops of Peppermint essential oil on the abdomen, place a drop on the tip of the tongue or wrists, or inhale to soothe minor stomach discomfort associated with travel.

7. For creepy crawly pests such as Silverfish and Centipedes, place several drops of Peppermint Essential Oil in places that collect moisture: basements, under cabinets, or in garages.

8. To stop ants in their tracks, wipe your cabinets with a damp sponge and 6-8 drops of Peppermint essential oil. Place several drops on windowsills, along woodwork or in corners

of kitchen countertop. You can also dilute 1:1 with water in a spray bottle and use as needed. Reapply in 2-3 weeks.

9. Uninvited guests, such as mice hate Peppermint essential oil. Add several drops of Peppermint in places where you suspect mice have been.

10. For indigestion or upset stomach, place one drop of Peppermint essential oil in 1/2 glass of water to sip slowly to aid digestion.

11. Bad sunburn? Add 6-8 drops of Peppermint essential oil in the bath to cool the body in summer. It is also great in the winter for skin protection.

12. To help reduce a fever, sponge the body down with cool water that contains one drop of Eucalyptus, Peppermint, and Lavender essential oil each. Or, just two drops of Peppermint essential oil.

13. Stay alert behind the wheel. Place 2 drops of Peppermint essential oil on a tissue and place in front of your car's air vent to keep you mentally alert.

14. Try dabbing a few drops of Peppermint essential oil on your face every night for the treatment of acne, pimples, insect stings, eczema and other skin infections.

15. Peppermint essential oil works great as a natural herbicide. Spray on unwanted weeds in the garden.

16. Give your feet a break! The menthol derivatives in Peppermint essential oil have traditionally been used in foot oils because of their healing smell and ability to kill bacteria and fungi. It will relax muscles, while the plant chemicals in them kill a wide range of germs and bacteria commonly found on the feet causing foot odor.

17. Massage several drops of Peppermint essential oil for an invigorating foot scrub. Combine with Lavender essential oil for a soothing massage.

18. Try Peppermint essential oil for spasms and to help reduce pain and swelling.

19. For bursitis, combine Peppermint essential oil with a carrier oil and massage in.

20. Peppermint Essential oil can be infused into chocolates or any other sweets by placing loose chocolates in a box, then placing a piece of absorbent paper with a drop of Peppermint essential oil on it. Cover and sit for a couple of days.

21. Make your own refreshing cup of Peppermint Tea, by placing a drop of Peppermint essential oil in a cup of hot tea.

22. Combine Peppermint essential oil with Lavender to help prevent colds and flu. Use only a couple of drops in a bath, massage oil or for inhalation.

23. For a deep facial cleanse, add a drop or two of Peppermint essential oil to your facial scrub or cleanser.

24. Peppermint essential oil detoxifies the liver and is an effective treatment for indigestion, irritated colon, and odorous intestinal gas.

25. Peppermint essential oil inhibits the further progress of herpes virus. Drink two cups of warm Peppermint tea during the periods when the virus is most active.

Clove Bud Essential Oil

From the Maluku Islands, known as present day Indonesia's Spice Islands comes the Clove tree, brought to the Middle East and into Europe well before the first century. During the late 1400's, the Portuguese cornered the Clove market, assuming control of the Maluku Islands. Spain unwilling to violate a treaty with Portugal, explored new ocean routes to the West Indies to obtain Clove, which led to the discovery of the New World by Christopher Columbus in 1492.

Clove Bud essential oil is distilled from the *Syzgium aromaticum* tree, a slender evergreen that can grow up to about 36 feet. The gray barked tree has shiny dark green elliptical shaped fragrant leaves. It thrives in lush tropical environments close to the ocean. Buds appear at the beginning of the rainy season. When they change to a bright red, this signals they are ready for harvest and are beaten from the tree and dried. One kilogram (2.2 lbs) of dried Clove buds yields about 150 ml (1/4 pint) of light golden yellow oil that has a medium to strong spicy rich aroma.

The word Clove is the Latin word, *Clavus*, meaning, "nail" because of the shaft of the bud resembling a nail. It is renown among the Chinese and Indian people for its medicinal value. Clove and Nutmeg also was considered very valuable in Europe during the 16th and 17th century. And no wonder since Clove relieves dental pain, toothaches, mouth ulcers, and sore gums, while its odor helps to neutralize bad breath. Today, it is frequently added to toothpastes and mouthwashes. It has also been found to help with other health problems like indigestion, coughs, asthma, headaches and blood impurities.

Alternative Medicine and Natural Remedies online forum reports, "This oil is high in Eugenol, a natural compound that successfully eradicates a myriad of harmful microbes including tuberculosis, oral & periodontal issues, scabies, parasites, wounds, cancer, autoimmune, Fibromyalgia, all respiratory concerns, cystitis, diarrhea, amoebic dysentery, fatigue, thyroid malfunction, bacterial colitis & ulcers, lymphoma, warts, viral hepatitis, neuritis, chronic skin disorders, insect bites, snoring & excellent for removing toxic chemical build up internally." Clove essential oil is also antimicrobial, antifungal, antiseptic, antiviral, and aphrodisiac with stimulating properties.

Because of its antiseptic quality, it is effective for treating wounds, cuts, athlete's foot, fungal infections, bruises and acne. It is also very good for insect bites and stings and a number of other conditions. Clove essential oil has been found to be helpful when battling flu's and colds and is used by dentists and in many dental products.

While Clove Bud embellishes itself with stimulating properties, it encourages sleep with motivating dreams and creates a sense of well-being and courage.

Used as a spice in cuisines all around the world, Clove is a treasure trove of minerals like Calcium, iron, sodium, hydrochloric acid, phosphorous, potassium and Vitamins A and C. It is the most powerful known antioxidant, coming in at approximately 10,800,000, the highest rating on the ORAC scale of any organic substance. Clove stops free radical damage dead in their tracks.

Clove Bud essential oil blends well with Lemon, Peppermint and Rosemary essential oils.

Plant Origin: Madagascar, Spice Islands

Medicinal Properties: Highly antimicrobial, antiseptic, analgesic, bactericidal, antioxidant, hemostatic (blood thinning), anti-inflammatory, pain killer, carminative, stimulant, antispasmodic and sedative.

Traditional Uses: Archaeologists have dated a ceramic container of Clove found in Syria to approximately 1721 B.C. and Chinese medical journals dating back to 400 B.C. mention Clove. One record from 200 B.C. tells of Roman Courtiers keeping clove in his mouth to keep from offending the Emperor from bad breath. Eugenol, the main constituent of Clove Bud is used by dentists to numb the gums. There is evidence that a solution containing .05% of Clove Bud Essential Oil was able to kill the bacteria, tuberculosis bacillus. Research by Jean Valnet, M.D., presented evidence that Clove Bud oil can aid in the prevention of contagious disease. Clove's powerful properties enables it to be for the sterilization of surgical instruments.

Other Uses: Clove essential oil can treat arthritis, acne, bacterial colitis, cataracts, bronchitis, cholera, cystitis, dermatitis, diabetes, diarrhea, dysentery, fatigue, halitosis, headaches, hypertension, insect bites, lymphoma, nausea, neuritis, rheumatism, viral hepatitis, and warts. It is also beneficial for intestinal parasites, tuberculosis, respiratory infections, pain, toothache, Fibromyalgia, scabies, and infected wounds. Clove treats and prevents infectious diseases, arthritis, dental infections, acne, fatigue, thyroid, dysfunction, sinusitis, skin cancer, chronic skin disease, bacterial colitis, and cold sores. Clove is good for Crohn's disease and low immunity. It possesses hormonal qualities, so it is good for thyroid imbalances.

Application: Diffuse. Apply topically, diluted with a carrier oil. A couple of drops can be added to water and gargle with the solution. For dental problems apply a few drops to a cotton swab and apply to trouble area. Clove is also good to help break nicotine addiction. Just apply one drop to the tongue.

Note: Many inhabitants of the island of Ternate died from epidemics after the colonization by the Dutch in the 16th century, who had eradicated the Clove Bud trees.

Safety: Liquid may irritate eyes and skin. Can be a sensitizer – use in dilution. Avoid if pregnant – abortifacient agent.

Safety Rating: C

Uses For Clove Bud Essential Oil

1. Add a few drops of Clove Essential Oil to a simmering pan to dispel household cooking odors.

2. Selling your home? Fill your kitchen with the aroma of Clove essential oil. Simmer a few drops of Clove essential oil in a pan of water on the stovetop.

3. Got a toothache? Clove Bud Essential Oil is a great choice. Place a couple of drops of Clove essential oil on gums for dental pain, toothaches, mouth ulcers, and sore gums.

4. Add a couple of drops of Clove essential oil to a candle at your next barbeque or outdoor party to repel mosquitoes.

5. Folklore says sucking on two whole Cloves without chewing or swallowing them helps curb the desire for alcohol.

6. To relieve nausea or stop vomiting, a few drops of Clove essential oil to a glass of water to drink. If not possible to get patient to drink, try one drop of Clove essential oil on the tongue.

7. Clove essential oil is effective against strep, staph and pneumomocci bacterias. Use diluted in a spray for the throat.

8. Ugly cold sore? Apply a drop of Clove essential oil or use in a bath.

9. For shingles, Clove essential oil helps topically or in a bath.

10. Add a couple of drops of Clove essential oil into a massage oil to help relieve stiff muscles and rheumatic joint pain.

11. For chills, add a couple of drops of Clove essential oil to a bath oil blend.

12. Clove essential oil helps to stimulate digestion, restore appetite and relieve flatulence.

Lemon Essential Oil

Citrus Limonum tree, a small thorny evergreen tree grown in India, as well as Israel, Europe, Florida and California delights us with the zesty fruit of Lemon. From the peel or rind of the fruit, we obtain its invigorating light yellow essential oil that has a thin consistency, with a rich aroma.

During the middle ages, Lemon essential oil gained popularity for its therapeutic properties among the Greeks and Romans. It especially increased notoriety when the British began using the fruit to keep their sailors from contracting scurvy.

The health benefits of Lemon essential oil can be attributed to its stimulating, carminative, and detoxifying effects. Its wide range includes Lemon essential oil's capability as an antiseptic to treating stress disorders. In Japan, a study has shown that Lemon essential oil vapor has anti-stress effects by modulating both the Serotonin and Dopamine neurotransmitter systems. The study's conclusion stated that Lemon essential oil has both anti-anxiety and anti-depressant effects. Other research in Japan showed a significant improvement in mental accuracy for office workers inhaling the aroma. Another recently published study showed that Lemon essential oil actually limits the toxicity of scopolamine, which causes dementia and memory loss. Lemon oil actually prevented these effects from occurring.

Because of its good taste and low cost, Lemon is very popular in cooking and serves as a good source of vitamins, which strengthens the immune system and stimulates the white blood cells to better fight diseases and improve circulation in the body.

Lemon oil blends well with many other essential oils including Lavender, Tea Tree, Cinnamon, Peppermint, Eucalyptus and Rosemary essential oils.

Plant Origin: Italy, Israel, Europe and America

Medicinal Properties: Antibacterial, anti-infectious, antimicrobial, anti-rheumatic, antiseptic, astringent, antispasmodic, antiviral, antifungal, carminative, diuretic, disinfectant, febrifuge and hemostatic. Lemon helps the immune system, encourages white blood cell formation and helps with circulation.

Traditional Uses: Lemon essential oil contains constituents that affect the immune system. Research done by Jean Valnet, MD showed Lemon can kill bacteria's like meningococcal bacteria in 15 minutes, typhoid bacilli in an hour, Staphylococcus aureus in two hours and Pneumococcus bacteria within three hours. One drop of Lemon essential oil can kill Diphtheria bacteria in 20 minutes. It has also been effective against infectious diseases like, typhoid, tuberculosis, and malaria and sexually transmitted diseases like syphilis and gonorrhea.

Other Uses: Lemon essential oil has been historically recognized as a cleanser (astringent) and antiseptic, with refreshing and cooling properties. Research has shown Lemon essential oil to enhance the ability to concentrate and improve memory. Other uses for Lemon essential oil include: strengthens nails, removes gum, remove wood stains, oil, and grease. On skin and hair, Lemon is beneficial for its cleansing effect and for treating cuts and boils. Other uses include: anemia, asthma, insomnia, rheumatism, parasites, insect repellent, malaria, warts, herpes, shingles, hair disorders, fights fevers, respiratory infections, mental fatigue, varicose veins, cramps, acidity, upset stomachs, and weight reduction. Lemon essential oil's benefits include its ability to treat nervous tension, relieve stress, and anxiety and is also helpful in promoting good sleep.

Application: Diffuse or Inhale. Make a spritzer, by adding a few drops of Lemon essential oil and Peppermint essential oil to sanitize the air. Lemon essential is food grade so it can be added to food or water as a supplement.

Note: It is great oil for mental clarity infusing one with energy. It is great for promoting health as well as healing.

Safety: It may irritate skin or eyes and cause sensitivity on some individuals. Lemon is phototoxic and should be avoided prior to exposure to direct sunlight. If you are pregnant consult a physician before using.

Safety Rating: B, G

Uses For Lemon Essential Oil

1. For smelly shoes, place a couple drops of Lemon essential oil directly in the shoes, or dabbed on a cotton ball and placed inside shoes.

2. Place a few drops of Lemon essential oil on a cotton ball and place inside your vacuum cleaner bag.

3. Apply one drop of Lemon essential oil directly to a wart everyday until it's gone.

4. Add a few drops of Lemon essential oil to a spray bottle filled with water and spray throughout your house to freshen up.

5. Add one drop of Lemon essential oil to a soft cloth to polish copper with gentle buffing.

6. For cleaning out the refrigerator or freezer, add one drop of Lemon essential oil to the final rinse water.

7. For acne, try liquefying cabbage leaves with witch hazel then strain. Add two drops of Lemon essential oil. Use as a lotion.

8. To treat troubled skin conditions, dab a couple drops of Lemon essential oil to your face and leave overnight. Wash off with warm water the next morning.

9. Baby got the sniffles? Add 2-4 drops of Lemon essential oil to a vaporizer (diffuser).

10. Place a couple of drops of Lemon essential oil on cotton balls and leave in specific areas to repel insects.

11. Did you know Lemon essential oil has hemostatic properties? It helps stops bleeding and with its bactericidal properties, it makes a wonderful wash for scrapes and cuts.

12. To detox, use Lemon essential oil in a lymphatic drainage massage.

13. Add a few drops of Lemon essential oil to a massage blend to help alleviate varicose veins. It is also helpful for the circulatory system and cleanses the blood.

14. Add a drop of Lemon essential oil to counteract acidity for rheumatic conditions, gout, arthritis and digestive issues. Lemon essential oil stimulates secretions from the stomach, liver and pancreas and supports the production of white blood cells.

15. Lemon essential oil is useful in skin care to brighten the complexion for oily skin. It also treats wrinkles and brown spots.

16. Add several drops of Lemon essential oil to a burner or room spray to help prevent the spread of infection.

17. Place a drop of Lemon essential oil on your toothbrush with toothpaste to whiten teeth.

18. Add 6 to 10 drops of Lemon essential oil to a spray bottle of water and spray it all over your pet's body, especially head and behind ears to get rid it of fleas.

19. Got cockroaches? Spray Lemon essential oil on problem areas.

20. Dab Lemon essential oil on socks and clothing to ward off ticks.

Eucalyptus Essential Oil

Native to Australia, the *Eucalyptus radiata* tree grows to the majestic heights of 270 feet. Young trees are adorned with oval-shaped bluish green leaves, while the more mature trees are draped with long, narrow leaves bearing a creamy-white flower with a pale green bark. With its strong herbaceous scent, Eucalyptus essential oil is extracted from its branches, leaves and nuts expelling a soft wood undertone.

Eucalyptus ushers in a welcomed addition to every medicine cabinet for its ability to fight colds, flu and fever. Its widespread applications include the oil's healing effectiveness for skin ailments such as burns, blisters, wounds, insect bites, and lice. Eucalyptus has a wonderful effect on wounds-when exposed to air ozone is formed as an antiseptic.

Another of the many benefits of Eucalyptus essential oil is its ability to help with muscle and joint pain. When blended with a massage oil, Eucalyptus acts as an analgesic, relieving the pain caused by rheumatism, sprained tendons and ligaments, lumbago, stiff muscles and nerve pain.

Eucalyptus' therapeutic value extends to rejuvenating the body with a cooling refreshing effect. This essential oil helps with exhaustion and mental sluggishness and is effective against stress and mental disorders. No wonder it is such a popular ingredient in room fresheners, soaps, detergents and many household cleaners. It can also be found in many over the counter cold medicines.

Eucalyptus essential oil is a very strong oil so use caution when creating your blend. It works well with Tea Tree, Cedarwood, Cypress, Frankincense, Lavender, Lemon and Rosemary essential oils.

Plant Origin: Australia

Medicinal Properties: Anti-infectious, antibacterial, antiviral, anti-inflammatory, analgesic, antiseptic, antispasmodic, deodorant, diuretic, decongestant, expectorant, febrifuge and stimulant.

Traditional Uses: Eucalyptus is used frequently to deal with respiratory problems and its ability to combat viruses. A solution of Eucalyptus is used clinically to wash out operation cavities and Eucalyptus-impregnated gauze is used as a post-operative dressing. It is valuable for burns as it helps to form new tissue as the burn heals.

Other Uses: A blend of Bergamot and Eucalyptus has been found to be effective against herpes simplex. It is also good for nasal and sinus congestion, as it helps to dry up phlegm and combat the infection of sinusitis. It is also used for acne, endometriosis, vaginitis and bronchitis. It has also been found to be effective on burns, blisters, cuts, wounds, insect bites, bee stings, lice, sore muscles and skin infections. Eucalyptus essential oil helps to heal ulcers and diabetes. Like Clove Essential Oil, Eucalyptus helps with dental problems. It is effective against cavities, plaque, gingivitis and other dental related infections due to its germicidal properties. Some of the other health benefits for Eucalyptus include: respiratory problems such as asthma, coughs, and bronchitis.

Application: Diffuse, steam inhalation or rub on the area of need or on the bottom of the feet.

Note: Eucalyptus contains eucalyptol which is used in many mouth rinses and products used to help relieve colds and congestion. *Eucalyptus radiata* is preferred over *Eucalyptus globulus* because it is less harsh, easier to inhale and doesn't irritate the skin as easily.

Safety: This should be used in dilution. Liquid may irritate eyes and skin. Avoid if pregnant. Do not used on babies.

Safety Rating: C

Uses For Eucalyptus Essential Oil

1. Did you know Eucalyptus essential oil acts as a good fly repellent? Just apply several drops to a ribbon and place on window sills or hang near open window or door. Reapply as needed.

2. When planning on going outdoors, try adding several drops of Eucalyptus, Bergamot and Lavender essential oils equally. Apply to skin with a carrier oil such as Grape Seed oil as a insect repellent.

3. To bring a fever down, sponge the body down with cool water than contains one drop of Eucalyptus, Peppermint and Lavender essential oils.

4. Baby got the sniffles? Add 2-4 drops of Eucalyptus essential oil to a vaporizer (diffuser).

5. Use Eucalyptus essential oil as a decongestant by adding to a pan of steaming water and inhaling deeply.

6. Eucalyptus essential oil is great for relieving headaches. Carry in a pocket diffuser for convenience.

7. Use a drop of Eucalyptus essential oil to relieve insect bites or stings.

8. To relieve the pain of shingles, use Eucalyptus essential oil in a bath or in a local wash.

9. Create a room spray using Eucalyptus to clear the air and promote healing.

10. Eucalyptus essential oil acts as a diuretic. Add Lavender and Lemon essential oils with a carrier oil to create a blend to help lose extra water weight.

11. Eucalyptus essential oil is beneficial for all respiratory tract infections, sinusitis, coughs, and sore throats. It is also works well for typhoid fever, tuberculosis, and malaria.

12. Use a drop of Eucalyptus essential oil on a sugar cube or in honey in tea or water for its strong antiseptic and diuretic effect on the urinary tract and bladder.

13. Eucalyptus essential oil helps your body fight off black-heads. It has a cleansing effect that removes dirt and oils and leaves your skin clear.

Lavender Essential Oil

Indigenous to the Mediterranean region south to tropical Africa and to the southeast regions of India, *Lavandula angustifolia*, commonly called Lavender, carpets their landscape with its faded purple flowers. Their prized spikes when dried are used domestically in potpourris, hand soaps and for sachets to give clothing a fresh fragrance and to inhibit moths. Of course, the list of uses is growing as Aromatherapists that have tapped into the therapeutic power of Lavender essential oil consider it to be one of the most versatile oils available.

Long ago housewives washed their bed linens in Lavender water and made sachets using Lavender blossoms to place between their sheets when folding bedding and clothing. It was believed that a home filled with the scent of Lavender indicated a fresh, clean, well-run house – one which was considered inviting to come in and unwind after a long day. Possibly that is why an old wives tale states that a married couple who keeps sprigs of Lavender between their sheets will never quarrel. Another folk tale suggests that a maiden who slept on a sprig of Lavender would dream of her true love, too. Its no wonder Lavender was a garden favorite!

Its name, Lavender is derived from the Latin word, *lavandārius*, which comes from *lavanda* meaning "things to be washed." The Romans added Lavender to bath water to soothe, calm and to treat the skin, while the Greeks crushed and burned it to create a calming fragrant atmosphere. They named Lavender *Nard*, after the city Naardus, located on a canal between the Tigris and Euphrates River, in the Baghdad, Iraq area. As a hub for Jewish study, the bible records the use nard in the Gospel of Mark, calling it Spikenard. In the ancient Mishna a Hebrew passage refers to it as *Shibolet Nard*, naming it as one of the ingredients in the Holy Incense.

Lavender flowerheads have culinary value as well. Bees attracted to its nectar find Lavender to be a culinary delight for making premium honey, while Sous Chefs around the globe garnish fabulous dishes with Lavender giving it a flowery slightly sweet taste.

As a member of the mint family, its woody evergreen shrub grows up to three feet with muted green narrow leaves crowned with violet-blue flowers. Lavender essential oil has a flowery scent with sweet undertones that calms, revitalizes and lingers in one's memory. Considered a balancing oil, it allows the body to relax and wind down but it also boosts stamina and energy.

French scientist Rene Gattefosse found Lavender essential oil to rapidly aid in skin regeneration after being severely burned in a laboratory accident. Lavender essential oil is made of hundreds of compounds known as constituents, of which scientists have only been able to identify 200 and believe this only to be half of what is in Lavender.

Lavender essential oil is very versatile and blends with a variety of other oils. Because of its sweet floral undertones, it is a good oil to add to heavier floral oils, as it will lighten the aroma. Lavender blends well with Lemon, Rosemary, Eucalyptus, Peppermint, Orange, and Frankincense essential oils.

Plant Origin: France

Medicinal Properties: Analgesic, antidepressant, antiviral, antifungal, antiseptic, antibiotic, antibacterial, decongestant, hypotensive, insect repellant, sedative, and vermifuge.

Traditional Uses: Lavender is probably the most popular and widely used of all essential oils. As a "cure all," Lavender's healing properties acts as a balancer and normalizes the body functions and emotions. Commonly used by the Classical Greeks and Romans, the ancients perfumed their bathwater with Lavender and believed it tamed lions and tigers. In ancient times Lavender was the oil of choice in cleansing wounds and during epidemics it was used to disinfect and purify the air. During the Black Plague, a quaint village of Bucklersbury, England, the center of Europe's Lavender trade, suffered no losses because of Lavender's antibacterial and antimicrobial properties. During WWI it was used in hospitals to disinfect floors and walls.

Other Uses: Treats burns and promotes healing to prevent scarring, cuts and abrasions. Good for coughs, colds, and flu. Soothes the nerves and acts as a stress-reliever and nervine. Helps with nausea and acts as a carminative for the digestive system. Conditions of which Lavender essential oil is useful include: ulcers, acne, asthma, hair loss, insect bites, rheumatism, arthritis, muscular aches, cataracts, headaches, migraines, insomnia and stimulates the immune system. It is quite calming and relaxing and helps with mood swings, depression and PMS.

Application: Apply topically, diffuse, or inhaled. Lavender is safe for use on small children. May also be added to food or water as a dietary supplement.

Note: Lavender is a very versatile essential oil with multiple uses. Lavender blends well with Clary Sage, Rosemary Chamomile, Rose Eucalyptus, and citrus oils such as bergamot. With heavy floral blends such as Rose or Geranium it lightens the aroma.

Safety Rating: A

Uses For Lavender Essential Oil

1. To keep clothes smelling fresh, add a few drops of Lavender essential oil to a cotton ball and tuck in a drawer. This also helps to keep moths away.

2. If planning on being outdoors, try adding several drops of Lavender, Eucalyptus and Bergamot essential oils equally. Apply to skin with a carrier oil such as Grape Seed oil as a insect repellent.

3. Use Lavender essential oil to repel moths. Apply several drops to cotton ball and place in a closet or wardrobe. Lavender essential oil is also good for bee and wasp stings.

4. To ease headache pain, rub a drop of Lavender essential oil on the back of the neck.

5. To blend your own massage oil, add 3-5 drops of Lavender essential oil to 1 ounce of Jojoba or almond oil.

6. For cuts and scrapes, apply a couple of drops of Lavender essential oil as an antiseptic to promote healing.

7. For a restful night's sleep, place 1-2 drops of Lavender essential oil on your pillow before retiring.

8. To bring fever down, sponge the body with cool water that has 1 drop each of Eucalyptus, Peppermint, and Lavender essential oils in it.

9. To create a tranquil atmosphere in the office, diffuse Lavender essential oil.

10. Did you know that diffusing Lavender is helpful with anxiety and stress? A blend of Geranium, Lavender, and

Bergamot also helps to alleviate anxiety and depression. Add this blend to a room diffuser or add 6-8 drops to a bath.

11. For babies, create a gentle massage blend using Lavender essential oil to calm them. Add two drops of Lavender essential oil to two tablespoons of Sweet Almond oil.

12. To relieve inflammation, make a compress using Lavender essential oil.

13. For acne and other skin conditions, use Lavender essential oil (1:10) with water.

14. Lavender essential oil works great as a natural herbicide. Spray on unwanted weeds in the garden.

15. Rubbing Lavender essential oil on the feet has been shown to relieve depression, anxiety and stress, while relaxing the muscles. Studies show that Lavender also kills bacteria and fungi.

16. Make your own window cleaner by using a clean, empty spray bottle and filling with one part vinegar to one part water. Add 8-10 drops of Lavender essential oil which helps disinfects and smells wonderful.

17. Baby got the sniffles? Add 2-4 drops of Lavender essential oil to a vaporizer (diffuser).

18. For constipation, give your baby a warm bath to which you have added 1-2 drops Lavender diluted in 1 tablespoon whole milk.

19. For diaper rash, add two drops of Lavender essential oil to un-perfumed cream (that does not contain lanolin). (If your healthcare provider thinks the rash is caused by fungus, use 4 drops Tea Tree essential oil instead.)

20. To help relieve stress, add four drops Lavender essential oil to four teaspoons of carrier oil. Use as a massage oil before bed.

21. Use Lavender essential oils for all types of burns: sunburn, cooking oil splashes, hot motorcycle pipes. Use neat (applied to skin directly) on affected areas.

22. Place a cotton ball dabbed with Lavender essential oil in window sills to keep flies away.

Rosemary Essential Oil

Rosemary, an aromatic shrub called *Rosmarinus offici-nalis* c.t. cineole, is derived from the Latin which means, dew of the sea. It produces a pale-yellow oil which has a medium to strong aroma. The consistency of the oil is thin but has a strong, clear, penetrating, camphoraceous and herbaceous aroma. Its plant has a scaly bark and thin needle-like leaves and grows to about five to six feet. The Rosemary bush is in the mint family with cousins such as Basil, Lavender, Myrtle and Sage.

Most are familiar with Rosemary as only a popular culinary herb, yet in therapeutic essential oil form it holds powerful medicinal properties. In aromatherapy, Rosemary abilities range from stimulating cell renewal to healing respiratory problems and minimizing pain. Paracelsus, a renowned physician of the 16th century gave credence to the fact Rosemary strengthened the entire body and healed organs like the liver, brain and the heart.

Legend has it that the Rosemary flower used to be blue but changed to white when Mary, the mother of Jesus escaped to Egypt. The tale says that when she hung her cloak on the bush, the flower turned white and afterward became known as the Rose of Mary.

Rosemary when used regularly in hair care stimulates the follicles promoting longer, stronger hair. It slows down hair loss and graying and can be blended with Basil and Tea Tree essential oils to help with scalp problems.

This incredible oil is also helpful with skin problems and can be found in many beauty aids. It improves dry or mature skin, lines and wrinkles, and heals burns and wounds. It helps to clear acne, blemishes or dull dry skin by fighting bacteria and regulating oil secretions. It improves circulation and can reduce the appearance of broken capillaries and varicose veins.

Like Eucalyptus and Clove Bud, it is a disinfectant and is used in mouthwashes to aid in alleviating bad breath.

Rosemary essential oil helps to overcome mental fatigue, sluggishness, forgetfulness by stimulating and strengthening the entire nervous system. It enhances mental clarity while aiding alertness and concentration. Rosemary essential oil can help to cope with stressful conditions and see things from a clearer perspective.

For respiratory problems, the effects of Rosemary are unparalleled. When inhaled, it offers immediate relief for congestion, allergies, colds, sore throat and flu. It is also beneficial for other respiratory infections and bronchial asthma.

Rosemary essential oil blends well with Frankincense, Lavender, Sage, Cedarwood, and Peppermint essential oils.

Plant Origin: Greece

Medicinal Properties: Antiseptic, anti-infectious, antispasmodic, antimicrobial, antibacterial, anti-parasitic, antifungal, enhances mental clarity, expectorant, stimulant, supports nerves and endocrine gland balance.

Traditional Uses: The leaves of the Rosemary bush were burned to purify the air in hospitals for many years. Throughout the ages it was believed Rosemary kept evil spirits away. Genetic Resources and Biotechnology Division, Central Institute of Medicinal and Aromatic Plants in Lucknow, India reports the following: "After clinically evaluating the antimicrobial activity potential of the essential oil of Rosemary specifically for its efficacy against the drug-resistant mutants of Mycobacterium and Candida Albicans they reached this conclusion: Rosemary essential oil was found to be more active against the gram-positive pathogenic bacteria except E. faecalis and drug-resistant mutants of E. coli, compared to gram-negative bacteria. Similarly, it was found to be more active toward nonfilamentous, filamentous, dermatophytic pathogenic fungi and drug-resistant mutants of Candida Albicans."

Other Uses: Helps to improve concentration and good for the scalp and hair loss. Rosemary essential oil has the ability to stimulate cell renewal, stimulate hair growth, boost mental activity, and relieve respiratory problems. This oil has been found to be an effective pain fighter and helps with arthritis, sore muscles, headaches, muscle aches and rheumatism. It is best applied directly to the area of soreness. It is also good for relieving stomach ailments, like indigestion and stomach cramps. Rosemary helps to heals wounds, skin conditions, sore throats, colds, flues, fatigue, allergies, asthma, diabetes and other respiratory infections. It has also been found to be effective against some cancers. Other indications include, liver conditions, hepatitis, hypertension, hypotension, indigestion, myalgia and menstrual disruptions.

Application: Apply topically, diffuse, inhalation. Rosemary Essential Oil is food grade so it may be added to food or water as a dietary supplement.

Safety Rating: I, J

Uses For Rosemary Essential Oil

1. To ease headache pain, rub a drop of Rosemary essential oil on the back of your neck.

2. To promote alertness and stimulate memory, inhale occasionally during long car trips or while reading and doing paperwork.

3. Use 1-2 drops of Rosemary essential oil on your hair brush to promote growth and thickness.

4. Rosemary essential oil is a good addition to shampoo for hair care. Add 40 drops of Rosemary essential oil to 7-8 ounce (approx. 200ml) shampoo. For children and elderly, add only 20 drops. Rosemary essential oil helps to keep the scalp clean and prevents dandruff.

5. Create a bookmark for students by adding Rosemary essential oil to help them study and stay alert. Or, dab one drop of Rosemary essential oil on the wrists before taking a test.

6. Rosemary is reviving. Inhale to refresh the mind.

7. Add Rosemary essential oil to a massage blend to help relax tired, overworked muscles. Rosemary essential oil also detoxifies the lymphatic system.

8. To help encourage hair growth, make a hair tonic with Rosemary essential oil. It also helps prevent dandruff.

9. Diffuse Rosemary essential oil to help prevent the spread of airborne viruses and bacteria.

10. Use Rosemary essential oil as a liver tonic by adding a few drops in a morning bath.

11. Feeling confused? Inhale Rosemary to clear your mind.

12. For the heart, liver, and gallbladder, make a Rosemary essential oil tonic to help increase the secretion of bile and helps lower blood cholesterol. Add a few drops of Rosemary essential oil taken with water. Or, the best application is through the skin using full body massage or warm compresses directly over the liver.

13. To stimulate flow of menstruation, rub a Rosemary essential oil massage blend on the lower abdomen or add to bath oil.

14. Use Rosemary essential oil in a massage blend for involuntary muscle spasms or to enhance circulation.

15. Add a few drops of Rosemary essential oil to cotton balls to place in drawers. This will keep unwanted pests from nibbling on your clothes.

16. Rosemary essential oil stimulates circulation and thins the blood, which is beneficial for arteriosclerosis and high cholesterol. Regular full body massage is the best method as this provides the added benefits of increased circulation and relaxation.

Tea Tree Essential Oil

From the marshes of Australia, reaching heights up to twenty feet stands the *Melaleuca alternifolia* tree, from which Tea Tree essential oil is obtained. Its needlelike leaves from which this pale yellow oil is extracted, has a thin consistency, yet very strong medicinal aroma. History records that the Aborigines of the outback used Tea Tree oil for healing and rightfully so, as it is the best known for being a powerful immune stimulant against infectious organisms such as bacteria, fungi, and viruses. During World War II, every soldier and sailor was issued Tea Tree essential oil because of its effectiveness against tropical diseases and infected wounds. Cultivators and cutters were exempted from military service until enough Tea Tree was harvested for issue to GI's in the South Pacific.

Tea Tree essential oil's popularity continues, as can be seen in the surge of use in the plethora of products commercially. Tea Tree essential oil helps with colds, measles, sinusitis and viral infections. It is excellent for skin, hair, acne, oily skin, head lice and dandruff. Research has shown that when used before surgery, it strengthens the body and reduces the effects of post-operative shock. The Essential Oils Desk Reference states that Tea Tree essential oil is also helpful with the effects of radiation.

Tea Tree essential oil has stimulating effects on hormones secretions and boosts up the immunity, acting as a shield against infections. It can also be used in treatment of Tuberculosis. Because of its antimicrobial properties, Tea Tree kills and keeps away certain microbes (protozoa) which are responsible for causing Tropical fevers and malaria.

As an antiviral, the essential oil of Tea Tee can help rupture a virus' "cyst" (protective shell) and offer protection against such illnesses as the common cold, influenza, mumps, measles, and the chicken pox.

Acting as a sudorific, Tea Tree essential oil increases sweating and promotes removal of toxins like uric acid, excess water and salts from the body.

As an insect repellent, it works well keeping insects like mosquitoes, flies and fleas far away when applied to the skin directly. Tea Tree essential oil also kills intestinal worms like round worm, tape worm and hook worms when used internally under the care of a physician.

Tea Tree essential oil blends well with Cinnamon, Clary Sage, Clove, Geranium, Lavender, Lemon, Myrrh, Nutmeg, Rosewood, Rosemary and Thyme essential oils.

Plant Origin: Australia

Medicinal Properties: Antimicrobial, Antiseptic, Antibiotic, antibacterial, antifungal, anti-inflammatory, antiviral, balsamic, diaphoretic, expectorant, immune stimulant, anti-parasitic, anti-infectious, insecticide, decongestant, sudorific and expectorant.

Traditional Uses: Tea Tree has been used for thousands of years by the Aboriginal people and is the most "medicinal" of all essential oils with its powerful antimicrobial action against infectious organisms including bacteria, viruses, and fungi. Researchers have discovered the oil activates the white blood cells, the body's first line of defense. In 1923, carbolic acid was used extensively as a bacteria fighting agent, until Dr. A.R. Penfold found Tea Tree's antiseptic properties were 13 times more effective. With its cicatrizing properties, Tea Tree heals wounds faster, offers protection from infections and reduces scarring because of wounds, acne and eruptions. It is one of the most studied oils and research shows that it is12 times stronger than phenol, a common disinfectant used in hospitals.

Other Uses: Stimulant, good for Candida infection, thrush, nail infections, acne, athlete's foot, mouth ulcers, cold sores, immune system, aging spots, insect bites and stings. Good for easing cold and flu, asthma, and bronchitis. Also is beneficial as an urinary tract antiseptic, jock itch and other genital infections such as herpes; helpful in alleviating problems such as cystitis, yeast infections, trichomonal vaginitis, general vaginal infections, leucchorea. Great for cuts, abrasions, burns, boils, warts, chicken pox, sinusitis, dandruff, ringworm, tonsillitis, varicose veins, and hemorrhoids. Tea Tree has balsamic properties that help the body absorb vitamins from food more effectively.

Application: Apply topically, diffuse, or inhaled.

Safety: In occasional circumstances people can have allergic reactions to Tea Tree Essential Oil, from mild contact dermatitis to severe blisters and rashes. Undiluted Tea Tree Essential Oil may cause skin irritation, blistering and itching. Tea Tree Essential Oil should not be taken internally, even in small doses. It can cause impaired immune function, diarrhea, and potentially fatal central nervous system depression. Please note, the International Federation of Aromatherapists do not recommend that Essential Oils be taken internally unless under the supervision of a Medical Doctor who is also qualified in clinical Aromatherapy.

Safety Rating: D, H

Uses For Tea Tree Essential Oil

1. To make a natural flea collar, saturate a short piece of cord or rope with Tea Tree essential oil and roll up in a handkerchief and tie loosely around the animal's neck. Do not use Tea Tree essential oil on cats.

2. Tea Tree essential oil works as a powerful immuno-stimulant and helps in combating many illnesses and ailments. Diffuse or inhale.

3. For scrapes and scratches, apply 1-3 drops of Tea Tree essential oil to promote healing.

4. For burns or scalds, add a drop of Tea Tree essential oil directly onto the affected skin.

5. Tea Tree essential oil is a powerful antiseptic but be sure to dilute before applying to skin.

6. For athlete's foot, apply Tea Tree essential oil three times a day. Soak your feet everyday for 10 minutes in a Tea Tree essential oil foot bath (add 5 to 10 drops of Tea Tree essential oil in a bowl of warm water. Applying essential oil to the soles of the feet increases blood circulation, providing a refreshing and cooling sensation and reducing bacterial and fungal growth.

7. Baby got the sniffles? Add 2-4 drops of Tea Tree essential oil to a vaporizer (diffuser).

8. Diffuse Tea Tree essential oil to help prevent the spread of infection against bacterial, viral, and fungi.

9. To boost a weak immune system, massage Tea Tree essential oil into the skin (with a carrier oil) or use in bath oils. It is also great for glandular fever.

10. To alleviate the pain of shingles, mix Tea Tree essential oil with Aloe Vera gel and massage into skin.

11. Tea Tree essential oil is famous for its benefits for hair and scalp issues. Add a couple of drops to a tablespoon of shampoo when showering. Wash as usual.

12. To prevent a cold or flu, add several drops of Tea Tree essential oil to a pan of steaming water to inhale deeply.

13. Dab a drop of Tea Tree essential oil with a cotton ball for insect bites or stings.

14. Skin conditions and acne respond well to Tea Tree essential oil. Use a cotton ball to apply a drop of Tea Tree to troubled areas before bed.

15. For vaginal thrush, use Tea Tree essential oil in your next bath.

16. Place a drop of Tea Tree essential oil on tick bites. Remove tick before applying oil.

17. For boils, wash area then apply Tea Tree essential oil full strength with a cotton swab two to four times each day for four days. You may also want to apply a gauze pad saturated with the oil directly to the boil for up to twelve hours.

18. For mouth ulcers or canker sores, apply Tea Tree essential oil full strength directly to the sore several times until it heals.

19. For cold sores, place a drop of Tea Tree directly to sore for a week.

20. Got dandruff ? Add Tea Tree essential oil to your shampoo for dandruff, dry or oily scalp, and itchy scalp. Use 10 drops to an 8 ounce bottle.

21. For diaper rash, apply 2 to 3 drops of Tea Tree essential oil with a carrier oil to promote healing.

22. For ear aches, rub 2 to 3 drops of Tea Tree essential oil on the outer ear. Or, make a blend with 3 drops of Tea Tree and one teaspoon of olive oil and use a dropper to place a drop in the ear twice daily.

23. For toenail fungus, apply a drop of Tea Tree essential oil to the affected area.

24. For receding gums, gingivitis, plague or gum infection, swish a couple of drops with water around or apply a drop to your toothbrush and brush as normal.

25. To disinfectant laundry, add one teaspoon per load or to prevent transmission of fungal infections.

26. Dog got ear mites? Add 8 to 10 drops of Tea Tree essential oil in a tablespoon of olive oil. Use a small dropper and slowly drop inside ear, massaging the outer ear, allowing it to saturate the inner ear. Repeat twice a week.

27. Teen got pimples? Apply Tea Tree essential oil directly with a cotton ball three times a day until gone.

28. For splinters, soak affected area to soften skin, then apply Tea Tree essential oil directly to area. Use a sterilized needle or tweezers to remove, then apply Tea Tree essential oil again to clean.

29. For sunburn, mix one part of Tea Tree essential oil with ten parts olive oil or coconut oil. Spread over burned skin.

30. For mouth thrush in infants, apply one drop of Tea Tree essential oil to a cotton swab and lightly touch affected area. Repeat twice a day for two days.

31. Take a clean, empty spray bottle and fill with distilled water and add 20-30 drops of Tea Tree essential oil. Use spray to clean your exercise mat after a workout. Other oils you can blend with the water: Lavender, Peppermint, Cedarwood, or Eucalyptus essential oils.

32. For a vagina infection try soaking a tampon in 1 drop Tea Tree and 1 tbsp of yogurt. Yogurt helps to restore healthy bacteria. Also, massage the abdomen with a blend of Tea Tree, Lavender and Eucalyptus essential oils.

More Ways To Use Essential Oils

1. To freshen laundry, place a few drops of your favorite essential oil onto a small piece of terry cloth and toss into the clothes dryer while drying. Add 5 drops of essential oil to ¼ cup fabric softener or water and place in the washer.

2. Revive potpourri that has lost its scent by adding a few drops of your favorite essential oil.

3. Create your own natural air freshener by adding a few drops of essential oil to water in a spray bottle.

4. For holiday cheer, add a few drops of Clove or Cinnamon essential oil to a pan of water and simmer on stove or in a potpourri pot before guests arrive.

5. Create a romantic mood by placing a drop or two of Cinnamon essential oil into the hot melted wax of a candle as it burns.

6. To dispel household cooking odors, add a few drops of your favorite essential oil to a simmering pan of water.

7. Rub a drop of Peppermint essential oil on the back of the neck to ease headache pain.

8. Create your own blend of massage oil by adding 3-5 drops of essential oils to 1 ounce sweet almond or other skin-nourishing vegetable oil.

9. Freshen carpet by adding 8-10 drops of your favorite essential oil to a box of cornstarch or baking soda. Mix well, then let set for a day or two. Sprinkle over the carpet in your home, let set for an hour, then vacuum.

10. To make a natural flea collar for your pet, saturate a short piece of cord or soft rope with Tea Tree essential oil, roll up in a handkerchief and tie loosely around the animal's neck.

11. Freshen shoes by placing a few drops of essential oils directly into the shoes, or by placing a cotton ball dabbed with essential oil into the shoes.

12. Put a few drops of your favorite essential oil on a cotton ball and place it in your vacuum cleaner bag. Lemon and Lavender work great.

13. To keep rodents and roaches away, place a scented cotton ball with Peppermint essential oil in an inconspicuous corner of a kitchen cabinet. This also works great for adding a fresh fragrance to the kitchen and bathroom drawers.

14. To keep bathrooms fresh, sprinkle favorite essential oils directly on silk or dried flower arrangements. (You can also hide scented cotton balls in inconspicuous corners.)

15. Try making homemade soaps that offer therapeutic properties scented with essential oils. These will make wonderful gifts for friends and family.

16. Freshen up flower and herb sachets by adding a few drops of your favorite essential oil.

17. Fill your room with a wonderful fragrance by adding a couple of drops of your essential oil to a light bulb ring. (Make sure not to get oil inside the light socket.)

18. For your favorite hand washables, try adding a few drops of your favorite essential oil to the final rinse.

19. Create your own exotic perfume with essential oils. Add 25 drops of your favorite fragrance to 1 ounce of perfume alcohol, and then allow two days to age before use.

20. For uninvited guests to picnics such as mosquitoes, drop a few drops of Eucalyptus essential oil on the melted wax of a candle or place a few drops on the Bar-B-Q hot coals.

21. Apply 1 drop of Lemon essential oil directly to a wart as an effective means of elimination. Apply the essential oil daily until the wart is gone.

22. Rosemary essential oil promotes alertness and stimulates memory. Inhale occasionally during long car trips, while reading and/or studying.

23. Home for sale? Fragrance matters. Fill the kitchen area with the aroma of spices such as Cinnamon and Clove. Simmer a few drops of the essential oils. Lemon essential oil sprinkled throughout the home on dried flower arrangements or on a door wreath creates a warm, cheerful and inviting mood.

24. Add Cinnamon essential oil to furniture polish and wipe down the wood.

25. Add essential oils to paper products, such as napkins and hand towels.

26. Infuse stationery and bookmarks with your favorite essential oil. Place drops of your essential oils on paper and put them in a plastic bag. Seal it and leave overnight to infuse the aroma. Send only good news in perfumed letters.

27. Padded and decorative hangers make more memorable gifts simply by putting a couple of drops of essential oils on

them. Be sure to pray for the recipient before giving them the gift.

28. Lavender and Peppermint essential oil helps to soothe away the effects of overindulges.

29. Make your own blend with essential oils for a soothing bath. Add 6-8 drops of your blend in a bath.

30. All of the essential oils, including Eucalyptus, Cinnamon, Clove essential oil make wonderful firewood oil. Drop approximately 2-3 drops of oil or a blend of your choice on a dried log and allow time for the oil to soak in before adding the log on the fire.

31. Sprinkle Rosemary essential oil on the outside of your window frames to deter flies and moths from entering.

32. For a restful sleep, place 1 or 2 drops of Lavender on your pillow before retiring.

33. When moving into a new place, use a water spray bottle containing Rosemary or Lemon to spiritually cleanse the atmosphere as you pray and plead the Blood of the Lamb over your home.

34. An ideal scent for the bedroom is Cinnamon essential oil.

35. Add 1 drop of your favorite essential oil to the final rinse water when cleaning out the fridge, freezer, or oven.

36. Use 1 drop of Clove essential oil on a washcloth-wrapped ice cube to relieve teething pain in children.

37. Add 1 drop of Lavender or Tea Tree essential oil to your facial moisturizer to bring out a radiant glow in your skin.

38. Place 1 or 2 drops of Rosemary essential oil on your hair brush before brushing to promote growth and thickness.

39. Add a few drops of Cinnamon or Clove essential oil to your diffuser when the flu is going around.

40. Don't be afraid to bring your essential oils to work with you. Many of your essential oils can create a calm working environment, and others will stimulate the senses and help give you mental clarity.

41. To help relieve tension, dilute 1 drop of Peppermint essential oil in 1 teaspoon of carrier oil, then rub on the back of the neck.

42. Give your pet a bath using essential oils if flea infested. Add a few drops of essential oils of Tea Tree essential oil, Rosemary essential oil, and Lavender essential oil in the bath water.

43. Place a cotton ball dabbed with Lemon or Tea Tree essential oil in sneakers or shoes to freshen. Leave in shoes overnight.

44. Add one drop of Lemon to your trash cans to keep fresh.

45. Tired muscles and aching joints? Add one part each of Eucalyptus essential oil to four parts Jojoba oil. Massage into sore muscles as needed.

46. To make your own perfume, add 25 drops of your favorite essential oil to one ounce of Jojoba oil. Let sit in a tightly capped bottle for two weeks before using.

47. Add fragrance to your bathroom with scented toilet paper roller. Place a few drops of essential oils on the cardboard

tube that holds the toilet paper. Every time it's spun, a fresh aroma will be released.

48. Add Eucalyptus essential oil to the laundry when you wash bedding.

49. For holiday parties or special occasions, fill up ice cube tray, dip a toothpick into your bottle of Peppermint, then swirl the toothpick in the ice cube tray to make Peppermint flavored ice cubes. In the summer, try using Lemon essential oil for iced tea drinks.

50. Lemon and Eucalyptus essential oils are effective against bacteria that cause staph, strep and pneumonia infections. A 2-percent dilution makes an effective vapor steam. Steam treatment carries essential oils directly to sinuses and lungs, and provides warm, moist air to help open nasal and bronchial passages. Cinnamon and Clove essential oils are beneficial as well.

51. Make a homemade pocket diffuser or inhaler by washing out an old chapstick tube and placing cotton balls inside it. Using a dropper, add several drops of your essential oil to the cotton then replace cap. Carry in pocket for quick access and use as needed.

Doc In A Box

While essential oils such as Clove, Lemon, Cinnamon Bark, Eucalyptus and Rosemary all have incredible benefits and healing properties individually, as a synergy blend they are even more powerful. Research at Weber State University has found when these essential oils are diffused they have a 99% kill rate against airborne bacteria. Other case studies concluded similar results demonstrating this combination of essential oils is proven to eradicate viruses and bacteria related sicknesses within minutes.

A legend is told of a band of marauders who stole from victims of the Black Plague in the countryside of France in 1591, yet never contracted the ravenous disease that wiped out ¾ of Europe's population. Upon their capture, the magistrate offered to spare their lives in exchange for their secret. The thieves, who were spice traders and perfumers, shared an old Egyptian alchemist's recipe of herbs and essential oils containing Lemon, Cinnamon, Clove, Rosemary and Eucalyptus. This information is said to be recorded within the Royal Archive of England.

Three recipes have been provided for making your own Doc In A Box blend. The first recipe is in an undiluted, concentrated form without a carrier oil. Please use caution as all essential oils should be diluted using a carrier oil or alcohol before applying to the skin.

Doc In A Box Blend Recipe 1:

Essential Oil	Number of Drops	
Clove Bud:	39	117
Lemon	33	99
Cinnamon	21	63
Eucalyptus	15	45

Rosemary	36	12
Bottle Size	5ml	15ml

Add essential oils to a glass bottle. Shake to blend.

Doc In A Box Blend Recipe 2:

1 Cup Jojoba oil (or another carrier)
1 Tablespoon Clove Bud Essential Oil
1 Tablespoon Lemon Essential Oil
2 ½ Teaspoons Cinnamon Essential Oil
2 Teaspoons Rosemary Essential Oil
2 Teaspoons Eucalyptus Essential Oil
Glass Container

Doc-In-a-Box Blend Recipe 3:

Use equal amounts of Eucalyptus, Rosemary, Cinnamon, Clove and Lemon, then mix with base of olive oil. For instance, when using a two-ounce bottle, place a tablespoon of each essential oil in the bottle. Then fill the rest of the space with olive oil. You can make a larger batch in a pint jar following the same proportion method.

Methods of Use For Doc In A Box Blend:

Diffuse: 10-15 minutes daily or apply to the bottom of your feet. Another convenient way to use your blend is to carry a pocket diffuser and inhale as you go about your business.

Ways To Use Your Doc In A Box Blend

1. When mopping floors, add several drops of your blend to your rinse water for the finishing touch.

2. Your blend does wonders in the garden too. Mix your blend with water in a spray bottle to repel insects on your flowers and plants.

3. Got a sticky price tag that won't come off? Use a drop of your blend to dissolve the gummy adhesive on price labels.

4. For bee and wasp stings, neutralize the toxin and relieve pain fast by placing a couple of drops immediately to the affected area.

5. Can't get to the dentist for an appointment? Hold off gum disease by placing a drop of your blend to affected gums until you can get treatment.

6. Your blend is great for reducing cavities too. Add a drop to your toothbrush when brushing. This will help maintain healthy teeth.

7. Got a toothache? Apply a drop or two of your blend to gums and teeth for pain relief.

8. Suspect there is mold in the house? Maybe down in the basement its musky? Diffuse your blend in your home or business to solve mold problems.

9. Add a drop of your blend to a glass of orange juice and drink to reduce phlegm and congestion.

10. For joint pain, apply your blend diluted and massage in for pain relief and to hasten healing.

11. Add a drop of your blend to your morning cup of tea for flavor and to maintain health.

12. To prevent infection in cuts and wounds, apply your blend diluted with a carrier oil to promote healing.

13. For sore throats, add a couple of drops of your blend with a tablespoon of water and gargle.

14. For bronchitis, apply your blend diluted with a carrier oil to the upper chest and throat for relief.

15. Place a drop of your blend on your thumb and apply to the roof of your mouth for a headache. This works fast.

16. For flu and cold protection, apply a few drops of your blend to the soles of your feet in the morning and the evening.

17. When you are stuffy and are suffering from lung congestion, add your blend to a pan of hot water and breathe in the vapors.

18. When cleaning pet cages, add several drops of your blend to a bucket of water with soap for a more eco-friendly green environment for them.

19. Add several drops of your blend to your dishwasher to sanitize your dishes.

20. Add 5 to10 drops of your blend to your laundry to make your clothes come out smelling fresher and cleaner.

21. If you are trying to quit smoking, place a drop on the tip of your tongue to help you curb the desire.

22. Got an ugly cold sore or canker sore? Place a drop of your blend on it to make them disappear fast.

23. For warts, apply your blend topically several times a day to make them disappear.

24. To help with pinkeye or other eye irritations, apply the Doc In A Box Blend diluted (1 drop to 5 drops carrier oil), around the eye. (Do Not Get In The Eye.)

25. Apply 1 drop of Doc In A Box Blend on your toothbrush to sanitize or place several drops in a cup of water to soak brush.

26. Create a bathroom spray using your blend for showers and toilets to sanitize and freshen.

27. For cleaning kitchen counters and greasy stovetops, place several drops of your blend on a moist sponge to scrub with.

28. Use your blend to clean and disinfect sickrooms.

29. Apply your blend to hands to remove stubborn, sticky substances like glue, oil or paint.

30. Add several drops to a bowl of water to wash fruit and vegetables from the grocery store.

31. Add several drops of your blend to the water in your vacuum cleaner/steamer to cleanse the air and disinfect the carpet.

32. Spray your blend along ant trails in the house to deter them.

33. Use your blend on a sponge to wipe chairs and furniture in school classrooms to cut down on sicknesses spreading.

34. When scrubbing floors or removing old varnish, use your blend to help prepare the surface for refinishing.

35. Add several drops of your blend to your cleaner when doing your upholstery. Make sure fabric is color safe.

36. Keep an extra bottle of your blend in the car for diffusing and cleaning the interior at the carwash.

37. Soak off burnt food in pots and skillets with a few drops of your blend. Then scrub away.

38. To sanitize trash cans, wipe or soak garbage cans with your blend diluted in a pail of water. This will help them smell fresh too.

39. For tough stains, add several drops of your blend on as a pre-wash stain remover before throwing into the wash.

40. For mold on walls and floor, clean using your blend undiluted to kill on contact.

41. For arthritis pain, rub your blend diluted with a carrier oil on sore joints for relief.

42. When a cold has gotten the best of you, add a few drops of your blend to a glass of water or juice to drink every three hours to stop it from worsening.

43. For herpes, place a drop of your blend on the tongue and/or a drop in a glass of water every day.

44. Keep your children healthy at school, by rubbing your blend on the bottoms of your children's feet before school every morning.

45. Diffuse your blend twice a day in your house before your children leave and when they come home from school to kill airborne bacteria or viruses. This will strengthen their immune system.

46. Mix your blend 50:50 with a carrier oil and rub on daily for relief of shingles.

47. When your dog or cat comes home scratched up, apply a drop of your blend on wounds to enhance healing.

48. Create a cheerful environment by diffusing your blend in the home.

49. To help increase mental concentration and work efficiency with the co-workers, diffuse your blend in the office or add to potpourri on your desk.

50. Ask your child's teacher to diffuse your blend in the classroom to reduce student sickness and absenteeism.

51. For coughs that don't seem to want to quit, add a few drops of your blend to a teaspoon of honey. This will be quite soothing.

52. For sinus headaches, rub a couple of drops of your blend mixed with a carrier oil over the bridge of your nose and breathe deeply.

53. Place a drop of your blend on pimples to make them shrink and disappear.

54. For laryngitis, place a drop of your blend under your tongue to restore your voice.

55. Diffuse your blend for relief of allergy symptoms. Carry a pocket diffuser with you of your blend to have on hand.

56. For Lyme disease, take a capsule full of your blend every day for relief of symptoms.

57. Carry a bottle of your blend on every flight to protect you from germs on the plane. Use wipes made with your blend to wipe pull down tray.

58. Diffuse and add several drops in the heat/AC vents of a hotel to rid it of airborne germs.

59. For cleaning bathtubs, mix your blend with your baking soda to replace other harsh cleaners.

60. For athletics' foot or fungus on the toenail, apply your blend undiluted to the toes and feet several times a day.

61. To relieve the itching of poison ivy, apply your blend diluted with a vegetable oil.

62. To remove permanent market stains, drop Doc In A Box Blend Oil Blend on a cloth and rub lightly.

63. Clean pierced earrings by dabbing a drop of your blend on with a cotton ball.

64. To help improve vision, rub a drop of your blend on your big toe before retiring.

Mental Clarity Blend

This one really does the trick when your mind tends to wander or you simply need a whiff of something to help you get through a mental task. Recent medical studies have shown Grapefruit essential oil to increase mental recall or memory by 25%.

What You Will Need:
5 Drops Peppermint Essential Oil
5 Drops Rosemary Essential Oil
5 Drops Grapefruit Essential Oil
1-Ounce Distilled Water
Spray Bottle

What To Do:

1. Fill spray bottle with distilled water. Add essential oils.

2. Shake well before spraying in the room. Use for helping with concentration or while studying.

3. Recipe Variation: Create an essential oil blend with out adding water and store in a glass bottle. Apply one or two drops to the temples.

Mental Clarity Blend #2

When you need an energy boost or need to oxygenate your brain, try this one.

What You Will Need:
½ Teaspoon Peppermint Essential Oil
¼ Teaspoon Rosemary Essential Oil
¼ Teaspoon Lemon Essential Oil
¼ Teaspoon Cinnamon Essential Oil
Small Glass Bottle

What To Do:

1. Combine all essential oils in a bottle. Shake to blend.

2. Inhale as necessary or diffuse for 10-15 minutes a day.

Migraine Chaser

Peppermint and Lavender essential oils make a wonderful combination for chasing the headaches away.

What You Will Need:
3 Drops Lavender Essential Oil
3 Drops Peppermint Essential Oil
1 Tablespoon Jojoba Oil (or another carrier oil)
Small glass bottle or vial

What To Do:

1. Combine ingredients in a small vial or bottle and shake to blend well.

2. Apply a couple of drops to your temples as soon as symptoms appear to ease your migraine headache.

Achy, Breaky Massage Oil

When the old body just isn't what it use to be and you're feeling older than you should, try a special blend of essential oils to soothe those aches and pains away.

What You Will Need:

1 Drop Clove Essential Oil
1 Drop Peppermint Essential Oil
3 Drops Lavender Essential Oil
3 Drops Eucalyptus Essential Oil
3 Drops Rosemary Essential Oil
3 Drops Orange Essential Oil
3 Drops Camphor Essential Oil
½ Ounce Sesame Oil (or another carrier oil)
1 Ounce Glass Bottle

What To Do:

1. Fill bottle with carrier oil, leaving space for the essential oils. Add essential oils and shake well before using.

2. If you do not have all of the essential oils listed, you can add other favorite essential oils in their place, or double another one listed (such as 6 drops of Eucalyptus, if Camphor is not available).

3. Have partner give you a back rub using your new massage oil blend.

Aches and Muscle Pain Formula

Gently massage into muscles to relieve pain.

What You Will Need:
2 Drops Lavender Essential Oil
2 Drops Rosemary Essential Oil
Massage Oil Base (carrier oil)

What To Do:

1. Add four drops of essential oils to 4 teaspoons of massage oil (carrier oil).

2. Massage into muscles for aches and pain.

Carpal Tunnel Relief

Whether your ailment is carpal tunnel, tennis elbow, or tendonitis, here's an easy recipe for instant relief.

What You Will Need:
¼ Teaspoon Rosemary Essential Oil
¼ Teaspoon Peppermint Essential Oil
¼ Teaspoon Eucalyptus Essential Oil
¼ Teaspoon Ginger Essential Oil

What To Do:

1. Combine all of the essential oils in a small bottle and shake to mix well.

2. When you are ready to use, pour a tablespoon of a carrier oil or massage blend into your palm, then add 2-3 drops of your blend.

3. Massage into skin.

Ease-Away Menstrual Cramps

Soaking in a warm bath with these essential oils can ease cramps.

What You Will Need:
½ Cup Epsom or Dead Sea Salts
5 Drops Lavender Essential Oil
2 Drops Peppermint Essential Oil
2 Drops Rosemary Essential Oil

What To Do:

1. Mix bath salts with essential oils.

2. Add to warm running water in bath to dissolve. Stir to distribute in bath evenly.

3. Soak for 20 minutes.

Pick-me-up Gel

Peppermint is a great pick me up for tired muscles.

What You Will Need:
2-3 Drops Peppermint Essential Oil
¼ Cup Aloe Vera Gel
¾ Teaspoons Cornstarch
½ Tablespoon Witch Hazel
Bowl
Pan
Small Container with a Lid

What To Do:

1. In a pan, combine Aloe Vera, witch hazel, and cornstarch. On medium heat, stir occasionally for five minutes making sure all ingredients are well mixed.

2. Allow mixture to cool.

3. Add Peppermint essential oil and stir thoroughly. Pour mixture into a clean container and cover with a lid. Keeps for four weeks.

4. Using a tablespoon of your gel at a time, massage muscles.

Sports Type Blend
Use this blend before and after exercise.

What You Will Need:
2 Drops Rosemary Essential Oil
1 Drop Eucalyptus Essential Oil
1 Drop Lavender Essential Oil
4 Teaspoons Massage Oil Base (carrier Oil)
Glass Bottle

What To Do:

1. Add all of the essential oils in a glass bottle then add carrier oil. Shake to blend.

2. Apply to body prior to and after exercise.

Joint Pain Relief

Eucalyptus is an effective analgesic used to relieve joint, nerve and muscle pain.

What You Will Need:
15-20 Drops Eucalyptus Essential Oil
15-20 Drops Lavender Essential Oil
1 Ounce Carrier Oil
Glass Bottle

What To Do:

1. Combine all essential oils and carrier oil in a small bottle. Shake well.

2. Massage in affected areas before taking a warm bath. Apply again after taking bath.

Minor Burn Relief

Use Lavender for immediate relief and healing.

What You Will Need:
2 Drops Lavender Essential Oil

What To Do:

1. Run cool water over burn for 5-10 minutes.

2. Apply two drops of Lavender (undiluted) directly on skin.

Anti-Gas or Nausea Relief

Find quick relief for tummy upsets with Peppermint essential oil.

What You Will Need:
1 Drop Peppermint Essential Oil
1 Teaspoon Honey or 1 Teaspoon Apple Cider Vinegar
Water

What To Do:

1. Add a drop of Peppermint to honey or apple cider vinegar.

2. Take with an eight-ounce of water to alleviate most gas and nausea.

Motion Sickness Relief

Carry this one with you for long car trips, or boat rides for sea-sickness. It also works great for morning sickness.

What You Will Need:
4 Drops Lemon Essential Oil
3 Drops Ginger Essential Oil
3 Drops Peppermint Essential Oil
Coarse Sea Salt or Himalayan Salt
Small Bottle 1ml or Vial

What To Do:

1. Fill small bottle with sea salt. Add essential oils.

2. Carry with you and sniff when you experience motion or morning sickness.

Cold and Flu Daytime Formula

Make this blend up in advance and store in the medicine chest.

What You Will Need:
2 Drops Peppermint Essential Oil
2 Drops Lavender Essential Oil
2 Drops Tea Tree Essential Oil
2 Drops Eucalyptus Essential Oil
Pan
Bowl
Water

What To Do:

1. Boil water in a pan. Pour water in a bowl.

2. Add essential oils. Let stand to diffuse in room.

3. Recipe Variation: Add essential oils to a cool-mist diffuser or vaporizer to diffuse in the room.

Cold and Flu Nighttime Formula

Make this blend up in advance and store in the medicine chest.

What You Will Need:
2 Drops Lavender Essential Oil
2 Drops Tea Tree Essential Oil
Pan
Bowl
Water

What To Do:

1. Boil water in a pan. Pour water in a bowl.

2. Add essential oils. Let stand to diffuse in room.

3. Recipe Variation: Add essential oils to a cool-mist diffuser or vaporizer to diffuse in the room.

Cold and Flu Relief

These essential oils work great as anti-viral oils and help support the immune system.

What You Will Need:
4 Drops Eucalyptus Essential Oil
3 Drops Tea Tree Essential Oil
3 Drops Rosemary Essential Oil
1 Tablespoon Carrier Oil

What To Do:

1. Mix all essential oils with a tablespoon of a carrier oil (any kind you like such as Jojoba, Almond, etc.).

2. Massage into upper chest and back. Place in a pocket diffuser for carrying with you or place three drops of essential oils on a tissue and inhale as needed.

Cold and Flu Relief #2

Here's another formula for fast cold and flu relief.

What You Will Need:
4 Drops Eucalyptus Essential Oil
4 Drops Scotch Pine Essential Oil
3 Drops Lemon Essential Oil
Bowl
Water

What To Do:

1. Add boiling water to a large bowl. Add essential oils.

2. Cover your head and bowl with a towel and inhale deeply for 5 minutes. Blend may also be added to a diffuser or vaporizer.

Sinus Relief Formula

Get instant relief from diffusing these essential oils when you feel the sniffles or a cold coming on.

What You Will Need:
2 Drops Peppermint Essential Oil
2 Drops Eucalyptus Essential Oil
2 Drops Tea Tree Essential Oil
Pot
Bowl
Water
Towel

What To Do:

1. Bowl water in a pan. Remove from heat.

2. Add essential oils.

3. Cover head and bowl with a towel then breathe deeply for several minutes to inhale fragrances. Keep eyes closed.

Stuffy Head Formula

Here's one to make in advance and have on hand during winter months.

What You Will Need:
10 Teaspoons Grapeseed Oil
5 Drops Lavender Essential Oil
5 Drops Eucalyptus Essential Oil
5 Drops Peppermint Essential Oil
5 Drops Tea Tree Essential Oil
Small Glass Bottle

What To Do:

1. Add all essential oils and carrier oil (Grapeseed) to the bottle. Shake well.

2. Use as a massage oil or apply to chest for protection from colds and flu. It can also be applied to feet before bed.

Cough Formula

Inhaling these essential oils will help ease coughs and bring quicker recovery.

What You Will Need:
2 Drops Lavender Essential Oil
2 Drops Eucalyptus Essential Oil
Pan
Bowl
Towel
Water

What To Do:

1. Boil water in a pan. Remove from heat.

2. Add essential oils.

3. Cover head and bowl with a towel and inhale deeply for 3-5 minutes. Keep eyes closed.

4. Recipe Variation: Add 2 drops of Lavender essential oil and 2 drops of Eucalyptus essential oil to a massage oil base and carry with you to apply to chest throughout the day.

Sinus & Chest Congestion Relief Formula

Keep these essential oils on hand for flu season.

What You Will Need:
2 Drops Lavender Essential Oil
2 Drops Eucalyptus Essential Oil
2 Drops Tea Tree Essential Oil
Towel
Pot
Bowl
Water

What To Do:

1. Boil a pot of water then remove from heat.

2. Add essential oils to steaming water.

3. Cover head and bowl with towel and inhale deeply for several minutes. Keep eyes closed.

4. Recipe Variation: Add essential oils to a room diffuser or vaporizer.

Cold Congestion Formula

These anti-viral and anti-bacterial essential oils will help loosen congestion, bringing fast relief.

What You Will Need:
4 Drops Eucalyptus Essential Oil
2 Drops Rosemary Essential Oil
2 Drops Lavender Essential Oil
2 Drops Tea Tree Essential Oil
1 Tablespoon Carrier Oil

What To Do:

1. Mix all of the essential oils, then add one tablespoon of your favorite carrier oil.

2. Massage into upper chest and back for relief. For convenience, carry essential oil blend in a pocket diffuser or place several drops on a tissue to inhale as needed.

Flu Buster

Diffuse this to chase those winter flu-bugs away.

What You Will Need:
4 Drops Eucalyptus Essential Oil
4 Drops Scotch Pine Essential Oil
3 Drops Lemon Essential Oil
Bowl
Boiling Water

What To Do:

1. Add steaming hot water to a bowl then add essential oils.

2. Cover head and bowl with towel and inhale deeply for 2-5 minutes.

3. Recipe Variation: Diffuse or use essential oil blend in a vaporizer.

Antiviral Spray

For those times when the bug is going around.

What You Will Need:
10 Drops Eucalyptus Essential Oil
8 Drops Tea Tree Essential Oil
5 Drops Thyme Essential Oil
6 Drops Lavender Essential Oil
2 Ounce Water
Spray Bottle

What To Do:

1. Combine all ingredients in a spray bottle. Fill the reminder of space with water. Shake well.

2. Use as needed or just add six drops of essential oil blend (without water) to a diffuser.

Flu Buster Spray

Having a spray bottle of this germ fighting antiseptic in your purse comes in handy when you are out and about shopping or in a place where water is not available for hand washing.

What You Will Need:
12 Drops Tea Tree Essential Oil
6 Drops Eucalyptus Essential Oil
6 Drops Lemon Essential Oil
2 Ounces Distilled Water
Spray bottle

What To Do:

1. Combine all ingredients and shake well to blend.

2. Spray to sanitize hands or to use on cuts and scratches. It can also be used as a room spray.

Four Thieves Vinegar

Here's one version of the ancient Egyptian alchemist recipe used by the thieves during the black plague.

What You Will Need:
1 Part Dried Lavender
1 Part Dried Sage
1 Part Dried Thyme
1 Part Dried Lemon Balm
1 Part Dried Hyssop
1 Part Dried Peppermint
1 Handful Garlic Cloves
Raw Organic Apple Cider Vinegar (unpasteurized)
Glass Jar

What To Do:

1. Place all dry ingredients in a glass jar.

2. Add Apple Cider Vinegar to saturate and cover herbs.

3. Place jar in a cool place and let sit at room temperature for 4-6 weeks.

4. Strain off herbs and collect vinegar in a clean jar and cover with lid.

5. To use vinegar, take a teaspoonful three times a day. You may also want to use as a salad dressing or marinade. Other uses include adding a teaspoon to bath water or making a topical spray for disinfecting kitchen or bathroom counters.

Athlete's Foot and Ringworm Blend
Try this, it works!

What You Will Need:
1 Drop Lavender Essential Oil
2 Drops Tea Tree Essential Oil
Grapeseed, Almond or Jojoba Oil

What To Do:

1. Add Lavender and Tea Tree to one teaspoon of carrier oil.

2. Apply with a cotton swab two to three times a day.

Foot Powder

Aromatherapy for the Feet.

What You Will Need:
1 Cup Cornstarch
1 Tablespoon Baking Soda
15 Drops Essential Oil (Peppermint, Rosemary, or Tea Tree)
Glass Jar with Lid

What To Do:

1. Mix all dry ingredients in a bowl. Add 15-20 drops of essential oils and blend in mixture.

2. Place powder in jar and shake well.

Foot Scrub

Exfoliate those rough places and leave your skin feeling soft and smooth again.

What You Will Need:
¼ Cup Dead Sea Salts
¼ Cup Sweet Almond Oil
10 Drops Essential Oil
Bowl
Glass Jar

What To Do:

1. Pour Dead Sea Salts into a bowl and add Almond oil. Blend well.

2. Add your favorite essential oil or blend to the mixture. Stir until completely blended.

3. Place mixture into a glass jar for storage. To use, scoop a small amount into your hand and scrub heels and feet in the tub or shower. Rinse.

Tea Tree Foot Powder
Keep your feet dry and odor free.

What You Will Need:
½ Cup Arrowroot (powder)
½ Cup Cosmetic Clay
2 Tablespoons Ginger
20 Drops Tea Tree Essential Oil
Large Jar with Lid

What To Do:

1. Combine all dry ingredients. Cover and shake to mix.

2. Add essential oil slowly, mixing in. Shake well.

3. Using a flour sifter or mesh strainer to sift powder, removing any clumps.

4. Store in a jar covered in a dark place.

5. Apply to feet and body as needed.

6. Recipe variation: Substitute 20 Drops of Lavender essential oil for Tea Tree.

Soothing Foot Bath

Oh, my aching feet! Here's an easy recipe that is cooling and refreshing.

What You Will Need:
10 Drops Peppermint Essential Oil
1 Teaspoon Jojoba Oil (or another carrier you like)
1 Cup Dead Sea Salts
Foot Bath
Small Container

What To Do:

1. Combine all of the ingredients in a small container. Let it sit for a couple of days.

2. To use, add 2 Tablespoons to a foot bath. Your toes will thank you.

Citrus Lemon Nail Care

Lemon is known for its antiseptic properties and has been used for centuries for hands and nails. It whitens and promotes healthy growth.

What You Will Need:
8 Ounce Spring Water
1 Tablespoon Aloe Vera Gel
10 Drops Lemon Essential Oil
Small Bowl

What To Do:

1. Mix all of the ingredients in a small bowl.

2. Soak fingertips for 10 minutes.

Clove Astringent Wash

Did you know Clove Essential Oil is a natural antiseptic and bactericidal herb? Clove Essential Oil can be useful in acne treatment as well. However, caution should be used, as it is not suitable for sensitive skin. Here's wonderful wash or toner, full off zest.

What You Need:
10 Drops Clove Essential Oil
Distilled Water
1-ounce Bottle

What To Do:

1. Fill glass bottle with distilled water. Add Clove Essential Oil.

2. Shake well before each use.

3. Use in shower as body wash. For treatment of acne, dab face with solution using a cotton ball.

4. Be careful to not get into eyes and other sensitive areas. May cause skin irritation.

Facial Mask for Acne

Acne plagues many teens and adults alike. Here's a natural alternative to the many drugs on the market that treat only symptoms.

What You Will Need:
1 Teaspoon Fuller's Earth or Kaolin Powder
2 Tablespoons Distilled Water
1 Teaspoon Base Powder
1 Drop Cypress Essential Oil
2 Drops Lemon Essential Oil
1 Drop Sage Essential Oil
Bowl

What To Do:

1. In a bowl, mix 1 heaping teaspoon of base powder with the essential oils. Add water and stir to mix well.

2. Apply to skin and leave on for 10-15 minutes then, rinse.

Acne Buster

Here's a simple formula for treating acne.

What You Will Need:
15 Drops Tea Tree Essential Oil
10 Drops Lavender Essential Oil
2 Ounces Jojoba or Almond Oil

What To Do:

1. Combine all ingredients into a dark glass bottle. Shake to mix.

2. Apply with a cotton ball to affected areas before bed.

Oatmeal Lavender Mask

Lavender is great for the skin.

What You Will Need:
½ Cup Ground Whole Oatmeal
6-12 Drops Lavender Essential Oil
Small Bowl

What To Do:

1. Grind the oatmeal in a blender or food processor.

2. In a small bowl, mix the oatmeal and essential oils and stir to blend. Add a few drops of water if needed to moisten.

3. Apply mask over the face. Leave on for 20 minutes then rinse. Use a warm cloth to soften mask and gently cleanse your skin.

Skin Tags Removal

While skin tags are considered harmless in the medical community, they can be physically irritating and embarrassing to those who suffer from them.

What You Will Need:
Tea Tree Essential Oil
Cotton Balls
Medical Tape

What To Do:

1. Clean the area of skin around the skin tag.

2. Pour Tea Tree essential oil onto the cotton ball and rub the skin tag.

3. Tape the cotton ball soaked with Tea Tree essential oil with medical tape.

4. Repeat the process several times a day until the skin tag loosens and falls off on its own.

Anti-Aging Formula

Keep your delicate skin smooth and nourished on your face with this facial oil.

What You Will Need:
½ Teaspoon Sage Essential Oil
½ Teaspoon Lavender Essential Oil
½ Teaspoon Rosemary Essential Oil
½ Teaspoon Rose Essential Oil

What To Do:

1. Combine all the essential oils in a dark glass bottle. Shake to mix.

2. To use, clean your face as normal then place a few drops on your fingertips and gently massage over your face and neck.

Cinnamon Toothpaste
When you run out of toothpaste, try this as a substitute.

What You Will Need:
2 Tablespoons Coconut Oil
1/3 Teaspoon Salt
3 Tablespoons Baking Soda
10 Drops Cinnamon Essential Oil
Glass Bowl

What to do:

1. In a glass bowl, mix all of the ingredients. Stir well until you have the consistency of toothpaste.

2. Use as normal. It will not foam up as a store bought brands, but will do the job in cleaning.

Super Brite Tooth Cleaner

Here's an inexpensive way to make your pearly whites sparkle and cure gum disease.

What You Will Need:
Hydrogen Peroxide
Baking Soda
2-3 Drops Lemon Essential Oil

What To Do:

1. Combine all of the ingredients to make a paste.

2. To use on teeth, gently rub on along gum lines and teeth. Brush as normal.

Trader's Moe Toothpaste

Tired of wasting a lot of money on expensive tooth-pastes? Here's one that you can easily make and you won't have to worry about chemicals like sodium lauryl sulfate in it.

What You Will Need:
3 Tablespoons Baking Soda
2 Tablespoons Coconut Oil
5 Drops Peppermint Essential Oil
Glass Bowl or Dish

What To Do:

1. In a bowl, combine all ingredients and mix well. Let sit for 5 minutes.

2. Use toothpaste as usual. This formula will not foam as normal toothpaste, but cleans just as well.

3. Recipe Variation: Substitute Cinnamon essential oil in place of Peppermint essential oil.

* Try this at Home: As a home remedy for acne, try putting this toothpaste on your pimple before you go to bed. It should help reduce swelling overnight.

Refreshing Mint Mouthwash
Fresh and minty - makes you want to smile.

What You Will Need:
6 Ounces Water
2 Ounces Vodka
4 Teaspoons Liquid Glycerin
1 Teaspoon Aloe Vera Gel
10-15 Drops Peppermint Essential Oil

What To Do:

1. In a pan, boil water and vodka. Add glycerin and Aloe Vera gel.

2. Remove from heat and let cool slightly.

3. Add Peppermint essential oil. Mix well.

4. Pour into a clean, plastic bottle with cap. Use as needed.

Herbal Mouthwash

This mouthwash help heals canker sores and mouth ulcers and alkalizes your mouth.

What You Will Need:
4 Drops Clove Essential Oil
2 Drops Myrrh Essential Oil
2 Drops Peppermint Essential Oil
1 Tablet Zinc
1 Tablet Folic Acid
16 Ounces Water

What To Do:

1. Let the tablets dissolve in the water.

2. Add Clove and myrrh essential oils to the mixture. Shake well.

3. Take some in your mouth and swish around then spit out. Do not swallow.

Dandruff Shampoo

This recipe is easy without spending lots of money on expensive hair products.

What You Will Need:
3 Drop Lavender Essential Oil
1 Drop Tea Tree Essential Oil
Baby Shampoo

What To Do:

1. In your palm take a spoonful of baby shampoo and add essential oils. Blend well.

2. Rub into scalp and let sit for five minutes. Rinse as normal.

Dry Shampoo

Here's a recipe for those moments when you need to freshen your hair in a pinch between shampoos.

What You Will Need:
¼ Cup Cornstarch
1-2 Drops Rosemary Essential Oil

What To Do:

1. Sprinkle cornstarch into your hand, then add a couple of drops of Rosemary Essential Oil.

2. Massage into hair and scalp. Allow it to absorb for a few minutes. Brush through hair. Repeat if necessary.

3. This is something you can take on a camping trip or when in a place where you can't use fresh water to shower.

Hair Treatment Formula

For strengthening hair at the roots, try this formula for 3-4 weeks.

What You Will Need:
3 Drops Rosemary Essential Oil
2 Drops Sage Essential Oil
3 Drops Grapefruit Essential Oil
1 Tablespoon Grapeseed Oil

What To Do:

1. Combine all essential oils and carrier oil.

2. Rub solution into roots of hair twice a week for 3-4 weeks. Leave on for 20-30 minutes. Wash as normal.

Hot Oil Treatment

Nourish your dry hair with this simple treatment. Olive oil not only nourishes your hair, but conditions and strengthens it.

What You Will Need:
½ Cup Olive Oil
5 Drops Rosemary Essential Oil
1 Plastic Bag (large enough to fit over head)
Jar

What To Do:

1. Pour olive oil into a jar then add essential oil. Replace lid and shake well. Let it sit overnight. Shake again before use.

2. Wash hair and rinse with warm water. Run jar under hot water to warm oil.

3. Apply a tablespoon of the olive oil blend and massage into scalp gently in a circular motion. Work oil into the ends of the hair.

4. Place the plastic bag over your head, securing tightly with a clip. Let sit on your scalp for 30 minutes.

5. Rinse hair, then shampoo as normal.

Hair Loss Treatment

This gentle treatment can be used on the scalp to treat bald spots.

What You Will Need:
2 Drops Cinnamon Essential Oil
4 Drops Cypress Essential Oil
4 Drops Geranium Essential Oil
2 Drops Juniper Essential Oil
5 Drops Lavender Essential Oil
3 Drops Rosemary Essential Oil
¼ Teaspoon Water
Dark Glass Bottle

What To Do:

1. Combine essential oils in a glass bottle and shake to blend well.

2. Place one drop of oil blend in your palm and add water. Rub on scalp in bald areas. Use at night before bed.

Hair Growth Formula

This recipe will stimulate hair regeneration and encourages growth.

What You Will Need:
10 Drops Rosemary Essential Oil
8 Drops Bay Essential Oil
7 Drops Cedarwood Essential Oil
2 Ounces Jojoba Oil
Shower Cap
Dark Bottle

What To Do:

1. Add essential oils and Jojoba oil to glass bottle. Shake to blend.

2. Apply to scalp then cover with a shower cap and leave overnight. Wash hair the next day.

Head Lice Removal

Here's a natural alternative to the chemical formulas for head lice.

What You Will Need:
7 Drops Thyme Essential Oil
4 Drops Tea Tree Essential Oil
3 Drops Rosemary Essential Oil
Hair Shampoo
Plastic Shower Cap
Bowl

What To Do:

1. In a small dish or bowl, add essential oils to two tablespoons of shampoo. Mix well.

2. Lather into dry hair and scalp. Cover head with plastic shower cap and let sit on head for one hour.

3. Rinse shampoo thoroughly and dry hair. Comb hair using a lice comb to remove nits and lice.

4. Repeat process in a week, then again in two weeks to insure complete removal of eggs and any lice that hatched in between time.

Body Care Recipes

Herbal Deodorant
This all natural eco-friendly deodorant works without all the harmful chemicals.

What You Will Need:
2 Tablespoons Aloe Vera Gel
2 Tablespoons Cornstarch
2 Tablespoon Baking Soda
2 Tablespoons Coconut Oil
10 Drops Tea Tree Essential Oil
10 Drops Rosemary Essential Oil
20 Drops Lavender Essential Oil
Travel Tin or Tub

What To Do:

1. In a small tin or tub, combine all the ingredients and stir well.

2. Dab a little on the fingertips and apply daily.

Rosemary Body Scrub

Invigorate your skin with this body scrub leaving a smooth, nice glow.

What You Will Need:
¼ Cup Sea Salts
¼ Cup Cornmeal
1/3 Cup Olive Oil (or another favorite carrier oil)
4 Drops Peppermint Essential Oil
4 Drops Rosemary Essential Oil
Bowl

What To Do:

1. Combine sea salts and cornmeal in a bowl.

2. Add warmed olive oil and essential oils, then add to the dry ingredients.

3. Use in the shower or tub. Rub on skin in circular motions, then rinse with warm water. Pat dry.

Minty Body Lotion
This tingly cream will revitalize your skin.

What You Will Need:
1 Cup Fresh or ¼ Cup Dried Mint Leaves
½ Cup Water
1/8 Teaspoon Borax
½ Cup Sunflower Oil
1 Teaspoon Coconut Oil
1 Teaspoon Beeswax
3-4 Drops Peppermint Essential Oil
Saucepan
Glass Measuring Cup
Container

What To Do:

1. Boil water with fresh mint leaves. Let cool. Strain off leaves.

2. Combine the mint water and borax. Mix well. Set aside.

3. In a glass measuring cup, add the sunflower oil, coconut oil and beeswax.

4. Place the measuring cup with the oils in the microwave for one minute or until beeswax is melted. Stir occasionally.

5. Take the mint water/borax mixture and microwave for one minute.

6. Combine the mint water/borax mixture to the beeswax mixture slowly and whip with a blender. Allow the lotion to cool completely so it can thicken.

7. Stir in Peppermint essential oil. The lotion will be a pale green color.

8. Pour lotion into a clean container with a lid. Use as normal.

Lavender Body Powder

This one will remind you of yester-years playing dress up at grandma's house.

What You Will Need:
1/3 Cup White Kaolin Powder
1/3 Cup Arrowroot Powder
1/3 Cup Cornstarch
8-12 Drops Lavender

What To Do:

1. Combine all of the dry ingredients in a blender. Add the Lavender essential oil and blend.

2. Put in a shaker jar or wide-mouth container with a powderpuff.

Private Signature Body Spray

Instead of purchasing expensive body sprays from department stores, make your own scented body spray using essential oils with aromatherapy benefits.

What You Will Need:
10 Drops Essential Oil (your favorite)
1 Cup Distilled Water
1 Tablespoon Witch Hazel
Spray Bottle

What To Do:

1. Determine what kind of body spray you want to create. For instance, a citrus body spray with Lemon invigorates, while a spray with Peppermint is energetic, yet cooling to the skin. A soothing spray with Lavender melts away stress and relaxes the body. Create your own "signature" blend.

2. Fill spray bottle with a cup of distilled water, witch hazel and essential oil.

3. Shake bottle well. Mist body after showering. After spraying in your eyes or directly on clothing that may stain certain fabrics.

Lemon Shower Gel

Start your morning right with a citrus body wash. Get an instant pick-me-up when you feel run down.

What You Will Need:
5-8 Drops Lemon Essential Oil
Liquid Castile Soap or Unscented Liquid Soap
Squirt Bottle

What To Do:

1. Combine liquid soap and essential oil and mix well.

2. Shower as normal.

3. Recipe Variation: Use Citrus Body Gel in a running bath to energize your body. Add one or two drops of Lemon essential oil to a moist washcloth and use as a compress on your forehead for ten minutes. Relax and be refreshed.

Liquid Antiperspirant Deodorant

Here's an easy recipe for a natural alternative for an antiperspirant.

What You Will Need:
¼ Cup Witch Hazel Extract
¼ Cup Aloe Vera Gel
¼ Cup Mineral Water
1 Teaspoon Vegetable Glycerin
2-3 Drops Cinnamon Essential Oil
2-3 Drops Lavender Essential Oil
Spray Bottle or Empty Roll-On

What To Do:

1. Combine all ingredients in a spray bottle. Shake well to blend.

2. Use as usual. This deodorant is good for athletics.

Rosemary Mist

Use this mist as an after-shower spray to stimulate your skin.

What You Will Need:
6 Drops Rosemary Essential Oil
1 Teaspoon Olive Oil
Distilled Water
Spray Bottle

What To Do:

1. Fill spray bottle with essential oil, olive oil and water. Shake well to mix.

2. Spritz on body after your bath or shower in the morning after you towel off.

Liver Detox

Doing a internal cleanse is important in ridding the body of toxins and functionally optimally.

What You Will Need:
30 drops Frankincense Essential Oil
20 drops Lavender Essential Oil
10 drops Clove Essential Oil
Castor Oil

What To Do:

1. Combine essential oils with castor oil.

2. Use as a compress over the liver five times a week for liver detox or liver cancer.

Pucker Up Lemon Lip Balm
Zesty and pumps up the smackers.

What You Will Need:
3 Tablespoons Sweet Almond Oil
1 Tablespoon Kokum Butter
1 Tablespoon Coconut Oil
1 Tablespoon Beeswax
1 Tablespoon Lemon Essential Oil
Small Saucepan
Small Tins or Tubes

What To Do:

1. In a small saucepan, combine all of the carrier oils. Melt over low heat until mixture is melted. Remove from heat.

2. Add a tablespoon Lemon essential oil and stir to blend. Pour into tins or tubes. Recipe makes approximately 3.5 ounce.

Peppermint Lip Balm

This refreshingly cool lip balm is great for the winter months for preventing chapped lips.

What You Will Need:
5 Tablespoon Jojoba Oil
1 Tablespoon Beeswax
1 Teaspoon Liquid Glycerin
5 Drops Peppermint Essential Oil
Small Saucepan
Tins or Tubes

What To Do:

1. Combine the oil and beeswax in a small saucepan. Warm until the wax is melted.

2. Remove from heat and while mixture is still warm, add the glycerin and essential oil and blend thoroughly.

3. Pour into your containers (tins, tubes, etc.). Recipe yields approximately 3 ounces.

Peppermint Balm (Recipe #2)

What You Will Need:
1 Tablespoon Beeswax Pellets
1 Tablespoon Cocoa Butter
2 Tablespoons Sunflower or Safflower Oil
6 Drops Peppermint Essential Oil

What To Do:

1. Melt beeswax, cocoa butter, and sunflower or safflower oils together in a glass measuring cup in the microwave for one minute or until melted. Stir.

2. Add essential oil.

3. Pour lip balm into ¼ ounce or ½ ounce tins or lip balm pots. Do not cap until lip balms have cooled completely.

4. Label and keep in a cool place. Makes eight ¼ ounce tins.

Bath Cookies

These are delicious for bath time, but do not eat.

What You Will Need:
2 Cups Rock Salt
½ Cup Baking Soda
½ Cup Cornstarch
2 Tablespoon Almond Oil
1 Teaspoon Vitamin E Oil
2 Eggs
6 Drops Essential Oil (Choose your favorite oil)
Bowl
Cookie Cutters
Cookie Sheet

What To Do:

1. In a bowl, mix all of the ingredients. Using the cookie cutters, create desired shapes.

2. Bake at 350 Degrees for 10-12 minutes. Allow to cool.

3. Use 2-3 cookies per bath. Store in an airtight container (use immediately because of eggs these are perishable). Makes a great gift.

Bath Fizzies
Create your own spa by making these at home.

What You Will Need:
2 Tablespoons Citric Acid (available at a pharmacy)
2 Tablespoons Cornstarch
¼ Cup Baking Soda
3 Tablespoons Coconut Oil (or almond or apricot kernel oil)
1-3 Drops Essential Oil (any fragrance you like)
3-6 Drops Food coloring (try mixing colors)
Bowl
Spoon
Waxed Paper

What To Do:

1. In a bowl, add the citric acid, cornstarch and baking soda and mix together.

2. In another bowl, mix the coconut oil, essential oil and food coloring together.

3. Slowly pour the liquid mixture into the dry ingredients and mix well.

4. Spoon a teaspoon of the mixture and shape into 1" balls.

5. Place the balls on a sheet of waxed paper to dry for a couple of hours, then, place each in a closed, airtight container.

6. At bath time, drop 1-3 bombs into warm bath water and enjoy.

Bath Bombs

These make nice gifts for wedding or baby showers.

What You Will Need:
1 Cup Baking Soda
½ Cup Cornstarch
½ Cup Citric Acid
15 Drops Essential Oils (use your favorite scents)
10 Drops Food Coloring
2 Bowls
Waxed Paper
Spray Bottle filled with Water

What To Do:

1. In a bowl, mix all ingredients except the food coloring.

2. Place a small amount of the mixture in a separate bowl. Add food coloring and blend.

3. Mist the salts with just enough water to help salts hold together (not too much to cause salts to start fizzing).

4. Pack salts in a soap mold, then turn over onto a piece of waxed paper. Allow to dry overnight.

Lavender Bubble Bath

Adding the fresh Lavender is what makes this bubble bath so special.

What You Will Need:
1 Bunch Lavender or Lavender Buds
1 Large Clear Shampoo (unscented, organic)
5 Drops Lavender Essential Oil
Wide-Neck Mason Jar (with lid)

What To Do:

1. Place Lavender head down in the jar. Cut to fit.

2. Add shampoo and essential oil. Replace lid and place in a sunny window for a couple of weeks. Shake occasionally.

3. Strain and rebottle. Use one tablespoon per bath.

Sparkling Bath Crystals

Here's an easy recipe for creating your own therapeutic bath salts. Customize these with your favorite essential oils.

What You Will Need:
¾ Cup Dead Sea Salts or Himalayan Pink Salts
¼ Cup Baking Soda
2 Tablespoons Citric Acid
20 Drops Essential Oil
Glass Bowl

What To Do:

1. Combine salts, baking soda, and citric acid together and mix well.

2. Add your essential oils to mixture and stir well. Let it sit for a week for salts to absorb fragrance. Suggestions for oil blends: Rosemary and Eucalyptus, Lemon and Lavender, or Peppermint.

3. Use ¼ cup of salts per bath.

Sweet Dreams Bath

Here's a sweet treat for a relaxing bath before bed.

What You Will Need:

2 Ounces Honey
5 Drops Lavender Essential Oil
Jar

What To Do:

1. Combine honey and essential oil in a jar and mix well.

2. Add 1-2 tablespoons to your running bath. Enjoy.

Lavender Bath Bombs

Make these for gifts and/or favors for a wedding or baby shower.

What You Will Need:
4 Cups Epsom Salts
2 Cups Sea Salts
2 Cups Oatmeal, Grounded
1 Cup Non-Fat Powdered Milk
40 Drops Lavender Essential Oil
Bowl

What To Do:

1. Make sure oatmeal is grounded fine, by using a coffee grinder.

2. In a bowl, combine all of the dry ingredients. Add the Lavender essential oil 10 drops at a time, then mix thoroughly. Repeat this four times, until all of the essential oil is distributed.

3. Use in bath or wrap in plastic and ribbon to give as a gift.

Fizzy Bath Salts
Put zest back into bath time.

What You Will Need:
3 Tablespoons Sea Salts
3 Tablespoons Baking Soda
1 Tablespoon Citric Acid
8 Drops Lavender Essential Oil (or another oil)
4 Ounce Jar

What To Do:

1. Combine all ingredients in the jar and shake to mix.
2. Add a ¼ Cup of salts to running water in bath.

Bath Salts Soak

This is great for relaxation or to detox.

What You Will Need:
10-12 Drops Essential Oil (your favorite oil)
½ Cup Epsom Salts
1 Tablespoon Baking Soda
Bowl

What To Do:

1. Combine all ingredients in a bowl. Pour in a hot bath while filling.

2. Soak for 20-30 minutes or until water cools.

Milk and Honey Bath

Soothe away dry skin with this milk and honey bath.

What You Will Need:
1 Cup Milk
1 Teaspoon Honey
1 Teaspoon Vinegar
2 Drops Peppermint Essential Oil
2 Drops Lavender Essential Oil
1 Teaspoon Olive Oil

What To Do:

1. In a large cup or bowl, add milk, honey and essential oils. Stir well.

2. Run a warm bath and add the mixture to bath. Swish around to blend. Soak and enjoy.

Zesty Shower Gel

Save tons of money by creating your own bath and body accessories.

What You Will Need:
½ Cup Unscented Shampoo
¼ Cup Water
¾ Teaspoon Salt
1-2 Drops of Peppermint Essential Oil
Food Coloring
Bowl

What To Do:

1. Pour shampoo in a bowl, then add water. Stir until well blended.

2. Add the salt, essential oil and food coloring (optional).

3. Recipe variation: Substitute Rosemary Essential Oil or another favorite essential oil in place of Peppermint Essential Oil.

4. Use as usual.

Lavender Bath Salts

Add color and decorative gems to make this one special for a gift.

What You Will Need:

¼ Cup Sea Salts
¼ Cup Epsom Salts
¼ Cup Baking Soda
18 Drops Lavender Essential Oil

What To Do:

1. Combine all of the salts and baking soda.

2. Add Lavender essential oil to the mixture (or another essential oil).

3. Use ¼ cup of salt blend per bath. Makes enough for three baths.

Candied Stripe Bath Salts

This makes a wonderful gift for a friend or family member. Try different fragrances and color. Mix and match — the combinations are endless.

What You Will Need:
3 Cups of Epsom salts or fine Dead Sea salts
3 Teaspoons of Sweet Almond Oil
9 Drops of Peppermint Essential Oil
1 Drop of red food coloring (more if you like)
Several jars with turn lids or cork seals
Ribbon for decoration
Gift Tags (optional)
Three bowls

What To Do:

1. Pour one cup of Epsom salts into each bowl.

2. Add a teaspoon of almond oil to each bowl.

3. Add one drop of food coloring to each bowl (any color you like). In one bowl you may want to add red coloring, in another bowl you may want to add a drop of blue food coloring, and so on. You may want to leave one bowl white.

4. Add three drops of Peppermint essential oil to each bowl. Stir to mix well.

5. Let salts sit for a few hours covered.

6. To create your candy cane effect, layer each color of salts with a layer of red, a layer of white, etc. until you fill the jar.

7. Replace lid on the jar and decorate with ribbon and tag.

Bridal Bath Salts

This makes a wonderful gift or favors for a bridal shower. Or, just something to have on hand for soaking in the tub and in God's presence.

What You Will Need:
1 Cup Bath Salts
3 Drops Rosemary Essential Oil
3 Drops Lavender Essential Oil
3 Drops Lemon Essential Oil
3 Drops Peppermint Essential Oil
4 Drops Food Coloring (choose 3-4 different colors)
4 Sealable Containers
Jar with Lid
Measuring Cups
Spoon

What To Do:

1. Place ¼ cup of bath salts equally into four containers with sealable lids.

2. Add 1-3 drops of Rosemary Essential Oil (or another fragrance) to the first container then, add 4 drops of red food coloring. Replace lid and shake to mix well.

3. Next, add 1-3 drops of Lemon Essential Oil to the second container then, add 4 drops of green and 2 drops of yellow food coloring. Replace lid and shake to mix well.

4. Add 1-3 drops of Peppermint Essential Oil to the third container then, add 4 drops of green food coloring. Replace lid and shake well to blend.

5. Finally, add 1-3 drops of Lavender Essential Oil to the fourth container of salts then, add 3 drops of red and 4 drops of blue food coloring and shake well.

6. On separate sheets of wax paper, spread out colored bath salts to dry for several hours. When completely dry, you are ready to layer each color in a pretty container. If you live in a humid area, you may want to speed up the drying time by spreading salts on a cookie sheet and placing in an oven on warm (or just a pilot light).

7. When completely dry, you are ready to layer each color in a pretty container. First, add the Rosemary, then Lemon, then Peppermint and finally Lavender on top.

8. If giving as a gift, add a pretty ribbon or raffia for decoration. You may also want to include a tag including each fragrant/color meaning: Rosemary (red) symbolizes covenant, (or if you chose to leave Rosemary (white) symbolizes purity, Lemon (light green) represents good life and health, Peppermint represents devotion, Lavender symbolizes lasting friendship and remembrance. Makes 8 ounces.

Suggestion: Try different fragrances and color combinations to reflect your faith or message.

Lavender Scented Bath Powder

Add your favorite essential oil to this simple recipe.

What You Will Need:
½ Cup Cornstarch
2 Tablespoons Arrowroot Powder
2 Tablespoons Baking Soda
3 Drops Lavender Essential Oil (or another essential oil)
Shaker or Container with a Lid

What To Do:

1. Combine ingredients in a bowl and mix well.

2. Let stand for a few days to dry, then sift through a flour sifter.

3. Pour into a shaker or container with a lid. Use as needed.

Garden Bath Tea

This tea for bath time makes a wonderful bouquet of fragrances for your senses.

What You Will Need:
1 Teaspoon Lavender Buds (dried)
1 Teaspoon Rose Petals (dried)
½ Teaspoon Lemon Balm (dried)
¼ Teaspoon Rosemary (dried)
1/8 Teaspoon Spearmint (dried)
4 Drops Lavender Essential Oil
2 Drops Rosemary Essential Oil
1 Drop Lemon Essential Oil
Empty Teabag
Bowl

What To Do:

1. In a bowl, mix all of the dry ingredients. Add essential oils, one fragrance at a time. Adjust to preference of scent.

2. Put into a paper teabag. Makes one teabag.

Lavender Scented Bath Oil

In a decorative bottle, this makes a wonderful gift.

What You Will Need:
4 ounces Almond Oil (or another favorite carrier oil)
2 Teaspoons Lavender Essential Oil
Decorative Bottle with cork or lid
Decoration (crystal beads, dried flowers, seashells, etc)

What To Do:

1. Using a funnel, fill a decorative bottle with almond oil, leaving a little space at the top, of an inch.

2. Add 2 Teaspoons of essential oil per four ounces of almond oil (or another carrier oil). Shake to mix well. Let it sit for 2 to 3 days before using.

3. Add decorative items to the container to make it appealing as a gift or match your bathroom décor.

Insomnia Soak Bubble Bath

Soak in this Lavender and Patchouli blend to relax before bed.

What You Will Need:
6 Drops Lavender Essential Oil
3 Drops Patchouli Essential Oil
1 Quart Distilled Water
4 Ounce Bar Castille Soap
4 Ounce Liquid Glycerin

What To Do:

1. Mix the soap, glycerin into the water and stir.

2. Add the essential oils and shake.

3. Add ¼ cup to ½ cup per bath and enjoy with soft music and candles.

4. Recipe Variation: For a "Wake Up Morning Bath" substitute 6 Drops of Lemon and 3 Drops Orange essential oils in place of Lavender and Patchouli essential oils. Or, for "Ole Man Winter Season Bath" use 6 drops of Eucalyptus and 3 drops of Peppermint essential oils in place of Lavender and Patchouli.

Kitchen Citrus Soap Wedges

These little soap wedges will brighten your kitchen with color and zest.

What You Will Need:
½ pound Transparent Melt and Pour Base
½ Tablespoon Coconut Oil
3 Drops Lemon Essential Oil
3 Drops Grapefruit Essential Oil
3 Drops Orange Essential Oil
Soap Mold (fruit wedges)
Orange, Yellow, and Green Food Coloring

What To Do:

1. Melt the soap base and coconut oil in the micro wave in a glass container.

2. Add essential oils and mix well. Using another bowl or container, divide the soap base and add the appropriate food color, then pour into the fruit wedge mold.

Appliance Cleaner

Here's an easy recipe that works as a degreaser and will make your appliances sparkle.

What You Will Need:

10 Drops Rosemary Essential Oil
¼ Cup Oil Based Soap (i.e. Murphy's)
2 Cups Water
Spray Bottle

What To Do:

1. Combine all ingredients in a clean spray bottle.

2. Shake well before using. Spray generously on appliances and let sit a few minutes. Wipe clean as usual.

3. Recipe variation: Use 10 Drops of Lavender Essential Oil or Lemon Essential Oil in place of Rosemary Essential Oil.

Appliance Cleaner #2

Here's another cleaner, especially great for stovetops and refrigerators.

What You Will Need:
4 Drops Lemon Essential Oil
1 Teaspoon Liquid Castile Soap
1 Teaspoon Borax
¼ Cup Lemon Juice
1/8 Cup White Vinegar
2 Cups Water
Spray Bottle

What To Do:

1. Combine all ingredients in a clean spray bottle.

2. Shake bottle to mix well. Spray generously on appliance surface then wipe off with a damp sponge. Wipe surface again using a clean cloth.

3. Recipe variation: Use 4 Drops of Orange Essential Oil or Eucalyptus Essential Oil in place of Lemon Essential Oil.

Microwave Sparkle Cleaner

Does your microwave still smell like the popcorn you made in it a week ago? Sometimes food odors get trapped inside the microwave, along with grease spills and splatters. Here's an easy way to take care of your oven and keep it clean.

What You Will Need:
5-6 Drops Lemon Essential Oil
¼ Cup Baking Soda
1 Teaspoon Vinegar
Bowl
Sponge

What To Do:

1. Mix baking soda, vinegar and essential oil in a bowl.

2. Use a sponge or clean cloth to apply paste and lightly scrub your microwave.

3. Rinse sponge and wipe clean.

Kitchen Sink Scrub

Use this cleaner in place of other harsh brands to scrub sinks.

What You Will Need:
1Cup Baking Soda
¼ Cup Vinegar
10 Drops Lemon Essential Oil
10 Drops Orange Essential Oil
Bowl

What To Do:

1. Combine all ingredients in a small bowl. Mix well.

2. Use as a kitchen or bathroom sink and tub scrub.

Citrus Glass Cleaner

Use this homemade spray to clean glass and polish mirrors. It will add a wonderful refreshing fragrance in every room.

What You Will Need:
4 Ounces Water
4 Ounces Apple Cider Vinegar
1 Tablespoon Borax
1 Tablespoon Orange Essential Oil
1 Tablespoon Lemon Essential Oil
Clean, empty spray bottle

What To Do:

1. Combine all ingredients in a plastic spray bottle then shake well.

2. Spray on surfaces and wipe immediately. Shake before each use.

Refrigerator Cleaner

Sometimes a box of baking soda just isn't enough to keep your refrigerator or freezer smelling fresh. Here's an easy recipe for a cleaner that will make it sparkle.

What You Will Need:
10 Drops of Peppermint Essential Oil
3 Tablespoon Baking Soda
½ Cup Water

What To Do:

1. In a bowl, mix water, essential oil and baking soda.

2. Clean as usual, wiping down shelves and door.

3. Recipe variation: Use Eucalyptus Essential Oil in stead for cleaning freezer.

Glass and Surface Cleaner

Here's another healthy way to use your essential oils and eliminate unnecessary chemicals from your home.

What You Will Need:
1 Cup White Vinegar
1 Cup Water
¼ Cup Rubbing Alcohol
10 Drops Rosemary Essential Oil
10 Drops Lemon Essential Oil
5 Drops Peppermint Essential Oil
Spray Bottle

What To Do:

1. Mix all ingredients together in a spray bottle.

2. Shake well before each use and use as normal to clean glass tables, mirrors and countertops.

Dishwashing Liquid

This soap is for hand washing your dishes. While it sanitizes your dishes, it will lift your spirit and helps strengthen your nails all at the same time.

What You Will Need:
16 Ounce Liquid Castile Soap (or mild dishwashing liquid)
10 Drops Orange Essential Oil
10 Drops Lemon Essential Oil
10 Drops Lavender Essential Oil
Empty, Clean Squirt Bottle

What To Do:

1. Combine all of the ingredients into a squeeze bottle. Shake well.

2. Use as normal for hand washing your dishes.

Kitchen Cleaner

Degrease your kitchen with citrus essential oils that make your kitchen smell great too.

What You Will Need:

8 Drops Lemon Essential Oil
15 Drops Orange Essential Oil
2 Tablespoon Liquid Castile Soap
1 Gallon Water
Bucket

What To Do:

1. Fill bucket with hot water.

2. Add essential oils and soap.

3. Mix well.

4. Mop or scrub floor as usual. No rinsing necessary.

Kitchen Counter Spray

Instead of filling our landfills with Clorox wipes intoxicated with numerous chemicals, try making your own kitchen counter cleaner. This is pretty enough to leave on the counter near the sink for quick clean ups.

What You Will Need:
15 Drops Lemon Essential Oil
15 Drops Orange Essential Oil
Beautiful glass bottle (wine bottle, olive oil, liqueur)
Spirit Pourer

What To Do:

1. You can use any old, fancy bottle you have available. Wash the bottle out thoroughly and fill with water. Add essential oil.

2. Recipe variation: You may substitute any of the essential oils for another kind of citrus oil such as Grapefruit, Lime or P`etitgrain.

3. Add spirit pourer to bottle (can be purchased at a kitchen store). Shake well to blend.

4. To use, pour a small amount onto a kitchen sponge or cloth and wipe down the counter. This will make your kitchen smell fresh and delightful.

Kitchen Floor Cleaner

Looking for a natural way to scrub those tough stains? Here's great home remedy for fighting grease. Give this vinegar formula a try.

What You Will Need:
20 Drops Tea Tree Essential Oil
2 Tablespoon Liquid Castile Soap
¼ Baking Soda
1 Cup Vinegar
1 Gallon Water

What To Do:

1. Fill a clean bucket with water. Add all of the ingredients, mixing well.

2. Clean your floor as usual. Rinsing is not necessary.

3. For stubborn stains, drop essential oil directly on the spot and wait a few minutes, then scrub off.

4. Recipe variation: Substitute 20 drops of Peppermint in the place of Tea Tree essential oil.

5. Recipe variation 2: Substitute 20 drops of Eucalyptus essential oil in place of Tea Tree essential oil.

6. Recipe variation 3: Substitute 15 drops of Orange essential oil and 5 drops of Lemon essential oil, in the place of Tea Tree essential oil.

Pine Floor Cleaner

Just like the pine floor cleaners from the store, except this one is all natural, which means it is healthy for you and your pets.

What You Will Need:
10 Drops Pine Essential Oil
5 Drops Tea Tree Essential Oil
5 Drops Cypress Essential Oil
2 Tablespoons Liquid Castile Soap
1 Gallon Water
Bucket

What To Do:

1. Fill bucket with hot water, then add essential oils and soap.

2. Mix well and mop as usual.

3. Rinsing is not necessary and you will be delighted with the pine fragrance on your tile floors.

Rust Be Gone Stain Remover

Why pay too much for cleaners that don't work. Get rid of those hideous stains with this easy remedy.

What You Will Need:
5 Drops Lemon Essential Oil
½ Cup Lemon (juice)
¼ Cup Baking Soda

What To Do:

1. Sprinkle stain with baking soda, then add drops of essential oil and lemon juice.

2. Let sit over night or several hours. Wipe baking soda solution away then rinse well.

3. Recipe variation: Substitute another favorite essential oil such as Orange in place of Lemon essential oil.

Kitchen Hand Soap
Have this soap on hand.

What You Will Need:
1 Cups Soap Flakes or Grated Soap
¼ Cup Glycerin
2 Cups Shampoo or Dishwashing Soap (unscented)
2-3 Drops Favorite Essential Oil
Bowl
Container

What To Do:

1. In a pan, mix the soap flakes, water and add two tablespoons of glycerin and set over low heat. Stir occasionally until the soap has dissolved. Store in a container.

2. In a bowl, add 1 cup of this mixture to the rest of the glycerin, shampoo and essential oil. Put into a quart container and store covered at room temperature.

3. Use ½ cup to tub while filling.

Fragrant Gel Air Freshener

Scented gel air-fresheners are great for the office, shop and home.

What You Will Need:
1 Tablespoon Salt or 10-15 Drops Grain Alcohol
2 Tablespoons Unflavored Gelatin (2 packages)
1 Cup Water
10-15 Essential Oils
Food Coloring
Salve Containers or Tins
Small Saucepan

What To Do:

1. Boil ½ cup of water, then add two envelopes of un-flavored gelatin. Stir to dissolve.

2. Add ½ cup of ice-cold water to gelatin mixture.

3. Add 10-15 drops of essential oil (any fragrance or blend you like).

4. Add 3-5 drops of food coloring.

5. Stir in a tablespoon of salt or 10-15 drops of alcohol, if used.

6. Pour gel mixture into 2-ounce tin containers. Allow to cool overnight (do not refrigerate).

7. To use, place open tins in the kitchen near a stove-top (not on a burner), or on the counter, in a window sill or in the car, etc.

8. Recipe Variation: Get creative by alternating colors in your tins by adding one color, allow it to cool for several hours then add another color, etc.

Apple Pie Spice Room Air Freshener

Make your kitchen smell like you have a fresh baked pie in the oven.

What You Will Need:
6 Drops Cinnamon Essential Oil
3 Drops Clove Essential Oil
1 Cup Distilled Water
Spray Bottle

What To Do:

1. Combine essential oils and water in a spray bottle. Shake to mix.

2. Use as needed.

Wood Polish

Why spend lots of money on furniture or floor polish, when you can do it yourself? Here's a simple one you can make.

What You Will Need:
10-15 Drops Lemon Essential Oil
2 Ounces Olive Oil

What To Do:

1. Fill a small bottle with olive oil and essential oil. Shake well to blend.

2. Apply wood polish by applying with a soft cloth and buff to shine.

3. Be sure to spot-check in an inconspicuous place to make sure your polish is safe to use on your furniture or floor. The olive oil feeds natural wood and the Lemon essential oil will make it smell fresh.

Recipes For The Bathroom

Bathroom Air Freshener

Eliminate odors and disinfect nature's way. This bathroom room spray will help you keep your bathroom clean by killing airborne bacteria and viruses on contact.

What You Will Need:
5 drops Cinnamon Essential Oil
5 drops Eucalyptus Essential Oil
5 drops Sage Essential Oil (optional)
5 drops Thyme Essential Oil (optional)
10 drops Lemon Essential Oil
10 drops Lavender Essential Oil
10 drops Tea Tree Essential Oil
Spray Bottle, 8-ounce
Distilled Water

What To Do:

1. Fill your spray bottle with distilled water then, add essential oils.

2. Shake well before each use. Store in your bathroom to use daily to keep it fresh.

Bathroom Air Freshener #2

Keep your bathroom clean from viruses and bacteria with this refreshing air spray.

What You Will Need:
5 Drops Lemon Essential Oil
5 Drops Cinnamon Essential Oil
5 Drops Eucalyptus Essential Oil
5 Drops Sage Essential Oil
5 Drops Thyme Essential Oil
10 Drops Lavender Essential Oil
10 Drops Tea Tree Essential Oil
10 Drops Rosemary Essential Oil
Distilled Water
Spray Bottle

What To Do:

1. Fill a spray bottle with 8-ounce of distilled water then, add all essential oils.

2. Shake this mixture well before each use. Spray every day to keep your bathroom smelling fresh and clean.

Bathroom Cleaner

Essential oils are some of the most powerful anti-viral and anti-bacterial cleaning agents around. Here's a great way to save money and create a healthy environment for the entire family.

What You Will Need:
2-3 Drops Cinnamon Essential Oil
2-3 Drops Eucalyptus Essential Oil
2-3 Drops Lemon Essential Oil
2-3 Drops Lavender Essential Oil
2-3 Drops Tea Tree Essential Oil
Distilled Water
8-Ounce Spray Bottle

What To Do:

1. Fill a spray bottle with distilled water and add essential oils. If you do not have all of the essential oils listed, you can substitute with another essential oil or double one. Do not leave Tea Tree essential oil out though, as this one is the most beneficial.

2. Shake well before each use. Spray in shower to keep clean and sparkle. Spray on toilet seat and wipe down. Use on surfaces to disinfect and doorknobs to sanitize. Your bathroom will not only look fresh and polished, but it will have a rich, refreshing scent you can only find with pure essential oils.

Tub-A-Dub Cleaner

Get rid of that ugly mold and mildew buildup in your bathroom using these essential oils.

What You Will Need:
1 Cup Baking Soda
20 Drops Tea Tree Essential Oil
20 Drops Lavender Essential Oil
20 Drops Lemon Essential Oil
Bowl

What To Do:

1. In a bowl, combine all ingredients and mix well.

2. Using a damp sponge, scrub tub or shower with cleaner. For tough stains or mildew buildup, leave on for 15 minutes, then scrub.

3. Recipe Variation: Just using the essential oils make your own "Fresh Shower Spray" by combining essential oils in a spray bottle with water. Spray shower daily after each use.

X-Mildew Formula

This formula helps fight fungus, mildew and molds in your home. Diffuse daily.

What You Will Need:
½ Teaspoon Tea Tree Essential Oil
½ Teaspoon Clove Bud Essential Oil
½ Teaspoon Lavender Essential Oil
Saucepan or Diffuser

What To Do:

1. Combine all essential oils in a saucepan of water or diffuser.

2. Use as needed. Diffuse for 10-15 minutes twice a day.

Herbal Disinfectant

Use this to clean counters surfaces.

What You Will Need:
10 Drops Thyme Essential Oil
10 Drops Tea Tree Essential Oil
¼ Cup Borax
2 Cups Water
Spray Bottle

What To Do:

1. Combine all ingredients in a spray bottle and shake to mix.

2. Spray on surfaces then wipe with a damp sponge or cloth.

Flu Buster Handy Wipes

Make these in advance to carry with you in the car or bus.

What You Will Need:
15-20 Drops Doc In A Box Blend
1 Cup Distilled Water
1 Roll Paper Towels (half sheet size)
Casserole Dish
Bowl
Quart Size Plastic Ziplock Bag

What To Do:

1. Cut or tear paper towel in half into 20-25 squares. Place towels in the bottom of a casserole dish.

2. Combine water and essential oil blend in a bowl. Mix well.

3. Pour essential oil mixture into the casserole, allowing the towels to absorb the liquid. Lightly ring the excess liquid off then fold in half and place in plastic ziplock bag or an empty wipe container. Use as needed.

4. Recipe Variation: For little hands, add ¼ cup of natural baby shampoo to your recipe to help get dirty hands clean.

Soft Lavender Scrub

Lavender makes this cleaner a joy to use.

What You Will Need:
¾ Cup Baking Soda
¼ Cup Powdered Milk
1/8 Cup Liquid Castile Soap
5 Drops Lavender Essential Oil
Water
Squeeze Bottle

What To Do:

1. Combine baking soda, milk, castile soap and Lavender in a squeeze bottle.

2. Add water to create a smooth paste. Shake to mix. Apply to surface then wipe with a damp sponge to clean.

Buzz Off Bug Repellent Spray

Here's a natural way to keep those pests from annoying you.

What You Will Need:
4 drops Eucalyptus Essential Oil
4 drops Lavender Essential Oil
4 drops Rosemary Essential Oil
4 drops Tea Tree Essential Oil
4 drops Lemon Essential Oil
4 drops Cedarwood Essential Oil
4 drops Pine Essential Oil
8 ounces Water
2 teaspoon Witch Hazel
Small, empty Spray Bottle

What To Do:

1. Combine all ingredients and shake to blend.

2. Apply to skin by spraying repellent on and/or rub in by hand.

Buzz Off Bug Repellent Skin Rub

1. Combine all of the essential oils listed in the Buzz Off Bug Repellent Spray recipe.

2. Add only 1 teaspoon of witch hazel and no water.

3. Rub directly on skin as needed.

Buzz Off Bug Repellent Oil

1. Combine all of the essential oils listed in the Buzz Off Bug Repellent Spray recipe.

2. Add only 1 teaspoon of witch hazel.

3. Instead of adding water, add 5 teaspoons of Olive oil.

4. Rub directly on skin as needed.

Citronella Soap

Makes a nice gift for the sportsman in your life.

What You Will Need:

1 Cup Grated Castile Soap
½ Cup Water
10 Drops Citronella Essential Oil
5 Drops Eucalyptus Essential Oil
1 Tablespoon Dried, Crushed Pennyroyal Leaves
Soap Mold
Non-stick Spray

What To Do:

1. Add grated soap, water, dried pennyroyal leaves and essential oils together in a large bowl. Using an electric mixer, whip the soap until it has doubled in volume.

2. Spray the soap molds with the non-stick cooking spray.

3. Spoon the soap mixture into the prepared molds, packing in as much as possible. If the mixture has cooled off and thickened, hand-mold the soap into large balls.

Poison Ivy Soap

This Camphor and Clary Sage soap is good to have on hand when a walk in the woods turns itchy.

What You Will Need:
2 Cups Melt and Pour Soap Base
2 Tablespoon Camphor Essential Oil
1 Teaspoon Clary Sage Essential Oil
Glass Container, microwave safe
Soap Mold

What To Do:

1. Melt soap base in microwave in a glass container. Add essential oils and stir until blended.

2. Keep soap wrapped or store in a cool place. It will be good for 18 months.

Nature's Hand Sanitizer

Take this with you on campouts, picnics, and day out-ings.

What You Will Need:
5 Drops Lemon Essential Oil
1 Drop Cinnamon Essential Oil
1 Drop Clove Essential Oil
1 Drop Rosemary Essential Oil
1 Drops Eucalyptus Essential Oil
1 Ounce Water
½ Teaspoon Aloe Vera Gel
Small Bowl
Small Container

What To Do:

1. In a small bowl, mix ½ teaspoon of Aloe Vera gel and one ounce of water.

2. Place one drop of Cinnamon, Clove, Rosemary and Eucalyptus essential oils in the bowl.

3. Add in 5 Drops of Lemon essential oil and stir well.

4. Store in an airtight container or travel-size bottle.

Sunburn Relief

Mist or rub on skin to take the heat out and promote healing.

What You Will Need:
10 Drops Peppermint Essential Oil
10 Drops Lavender Essential Oil
10 Drops Chamomile Essential Oil
1 Ounce Coconut Oil or Water
1 Teaspoon Vodka or Alcohol
1 Ounce Spray Bottle

What To Do:

1. Add essential oils and alcohol to the spray bottle. Shake well. Fill the reminder of the bottle with water or coconut oil.

2. To use, spray on skin for fast relief.

Sunburn Relief #2

If you've gotten too much sun and feel like your skin's on fire, cool down with essential oil.

What You Will Need:
1 Cup White Vinegar (or)
1 Cup Baking Soda
12 Drops Lavender Essential Oil

What To Do:

1. Run a cool bath and add either white vinegar or baking soda.

2. Add Lavender essential oil and swish around to mix well.

3. Soak in bath for 20-30 minutes. When finished soaking, apply a generous amount of Aloe Vera gel to skin for faster healing.

After Sun Spritz
Give your skin a drink after a day in the sun.

What You Will Need:
5 Drops Tea Tree Essential Oil
10 Drops Lavender Essential Oil
3 Ounces Distilled Water
Spray Bottle

What To Do:

1. Combine essential oils and water in a spray bottle and shake.

2. Mist skin with spritzer followed by a body lotion to seal in moisture.

Flea Control For The House

Sprinkle on carpet and then vacuum up to keep your home pest-free.

What You Will Need:
30 Drops Tea Tree Essential Oil
10 Drops Cedarwood Essential Oil
1 Cup Cornstarch
1 Cup Water
Spray Bottle
Bowl

What To Do:

1. Mix essential oils and cornstarch in a bowl and stir well. Sprinkle on the carpet and let stand for five minutes. Vacuum.

2. For the furniture, add essential oils and water in a spray bottle and spritz on fabric-safe surfaces. Penny royal essential oil may be substituted for Cedarwood, but care must be taken as it is not safe for pregnant women or cats.

Cinnamon Red Hots Soap

These little round soaps will remind you of the "little red hot" candies of yester year.

What You Will Need:

4 Ounce Melt and Pour Soap Base
10 Drops Cinnamon Essential Oil
1 Drop Red Coloring
Glass Container
Soap Mold
1 PVC Pipe Cap

What To Do:

1. Melt the melt and pour soap base in a glass container using a microwave.

2. Add Cinnamon essential oil and red coloring.

3. Pour soap into a mold and let set for several hours.

4. Cut soap into round shapes using a PVC cap.

Eucalyptus Fireplace Log

For the holidays, you can make fireplace logs using any of your favorite essential oils.

What You Will Need:
1 Drop Eucalyptus Essential Oil
1 Log

What To Do:

1. Apply one drop of essential oil to the log. Allow to sit for several hours so that the essential oil soaks into the wood.

2. Use only one drop of essential oil per log, per fire.

Scented Fireplace Cones

A nice addition to any fireplace is scented pinecones.

What You Will Need:
6 Drops Cinnamon Essential Oil
6 Drops Clove Essential Oil
Pinecones
Baking Sheet

What To Do:

1. Preheat your oven at 200 degrees or lower. Place a handful of pinecones in a single layer on a baking sheet.

2. Bake for 25 minutes. Keep an eye on these, since pinecones can ignite at high temperatures.

3. Let the pinecones cool completely, then sprinkle with a few drops of your essential oil blend. Place cones in a plastic bag and keep sealed until you are ready to use to light a fire. Place pinecones in a pretty basket next to the fireplace and toss into the fire one at a time.

Mint Chocolate Lip Saver Balm

This one not only is lip smacking good, it plumps your lips up to give them a fuller look.

What You Will Need:
3 Teaspoon Jojoba oil (or another carrier oil)
2 Teaspoon Cocoa Butter, prime-pressed
1 Teaspoon Beeswax
5-10 Drops Peppermint Essential Oil
Lip Balm containers or tins

What To Do:

1. Slowly melt ingredients in 30-second intervals in the microwave (or use a double boiler).

2. Let cool slightly then fill containers. Give to friends and family as gifts.

Mini "Stress Free" Aromatherapy Garden

A mini sand garden filled with aromatics is a great way to release stress and relax. This makes a great gift or for yourself to enjoy at the office.

What You Will Need:
Container (this can be a shadow box, glass bowl, etc.)
Sand (clean, colored if you like)
15-20 Drops Essential Oil (any fragrance you like)
Mini Rake, Rocks, Accents

What To Do:

1. Choose a theme for your garden. You may want a seascape theme using shells, or a more elegant look with a jewelry chest filled with jewels, or maybe a more eco-friendly natural look with smooth river stones, etc. The options are endless.

2. Choose a container that has low sides. This can be a jewelry box, glass dish, shadow box depending on the theme of your garden.

3. Fill your box with clean, colored sand. Now add ac cents such as shells, rocks, tools for raking the sand. Small miniatures tools and add-ons are available at craft shows or you can make your own.

4. Add several drops of essential oil to the sand, and rake in. (Option: You may want to use a small pot or container in your display to hold your essential oil instead.)

5. Play in your sandbox to release stress and breathe in the wonderful fragrances of your garden.

Creamy Rosemary Soap

Everyone loves the scent of Rosemary - even men. This is a great one to wake up in the morning to.

What You Will Need:
1 Pound Melt and Pour Soap Base
1 Cup Whole Milk
½ Teaspoon Rosemary Essential Oil
Non-Stick Cooking Spray
Cookie Cutter
Soap Mold

What To Do:

1. Spray your soap mold with the non-stick cooking spray.

2. Melt soap base in a glass container in the micro-wave. Add milk and essential oils and blend well.

3. Pour soap mixture into a mold and let sit for several hours. Push out of mold and use cookie cutters to slice soap into shapes.

*Rosemary Essential Oil is not recommended for individuals with epilepsy.

Romantic Cinnamon Night Powder

Sprinkle this powder on your bed sheets just before retiring.

What You Will Need:
½ Cup Cornstarch
½ Cup Baking Soda
8 Drops Cinnamon Essential Oil
Jar with Lid

What To Do:

1. Mix ingredients today until well-blended.

2. Add essential oil one drop at a time, making sure it mixes in.

3. Pour mixture into a jar. Punch a few holes in the lid (or purchase grated cheese shaker).

4. Sprinkle powder on your skin after showering and on your bed linens before getting into bed.

5. Recipe variation: Use ¼ Cup Cornstarch and ¼ Cup Rice Flour instead of ½ Cup of Cornstarch and Baking Soda. One tablespoon of Cinnamon powder may be used instead of essential oil.

Lavender Perfumed Lining Paper

Find a pretty lining paper and spice it up with a lovely fragrance.

What You Will Need:
Lining Paper
Blotting Paper
6 Drops Lavender Essential Oil
Large Plastic Bag

What To Do:

1. Cut lining paper to size and sheets together.

2. Add several drops of Lavender essential oil to blotting paper and place in a plastic bag with lining paper.

3. Leave paper in the bag for a week to absorb the fragrance.

Scented Bath Crystals

These are fun to make and decorate with.

What You Will Need:
Sea Salt or Rock Salt
2 Teaspoons Eucalyptus Essential Oil
8-ounce Clear Plastic Jar with Lid
Food Coloring (optional)
Bowl

What To Do:

1. In a bowl, add essential oil to sea salts. Add color if desired.

2. Pour into a container and replace lid. Wait several days before using.

3. This makes a nice gift. Decorate using a ribbon and tag.

4. Recipe variation: Adjust quantity of salts and essential oil for smaller jars or containers.

Room Spray

Freshen up your house with fragrant oils.

What You Will Need:
1.5 Ounces Distilled Water
1.5 Ounces Vodka
20 Drops Rosemary Essential Oil
4 Drops Peppermint Essential Oil
8 Drops Lemon Essential Oil
4 Drops Lavender Essential Oil
8 Ounce Spray Bottle

What To Do:

1. Fill the spray bottle with distilled water and alcohol (or just 3 ounces of distilled water).

2. Add essential oils. Shake prior to each use.

3. Mist each room lightly. Be careful to not use on fabric furniture.

Scented Get Well Cards

Add healing essential oils to your cards for friends and family who may be sick. This is a wonderful way to wish them well soon.

What You Will Need:
Get Well Card
1 Drop Cinnamon Essential Oil
1 Drop Clove Essential Oil
1 Drop Lemon Essential Oil

What To Do:

1. Choose your card then place one drop of any combination of essential oils or just one fragrance.

2. Seal and mail to recipient.

3. Recipe Variation: Use other essential oils such as Eucalyptus or Rosemary essential oils. Also, try doing this for the holiday and add Orange essential oil, or an Evergreen blend.

Scented Rocks

Make your own scented rocks to use like potpourri in a dish.

What You Will Need:
½ Cup Flour
½ Cup Salt
¼ Teaspoon Essential Oil (any fragrance you like)
½ Cup Boiling Water
Food Coloring

What To Do:

1. In a bowl, mix the flour and salt.

2. Add the essential oil and boiling water to the dry ingredients.

3. Add food coloring to create the desired color. Blend well.

4. Take a small amount to shape balls in different sizes to make stones. (Add more water if too dry.)

5. Allow to dry, then place in a dish or bowl to scent a room.

Ice Candles

Create your own signature design candles with your favorite scent.

What You Will Need:
1 Pound Paraffin
1 Taper Candle
6 Drops Peppermint Essential Oil
Glitter
Crushed Ice
Double Boiler
Empty, Clean Milk Carton

What To Do:

1. Melt the paraffin in a double boiler.

2. Cut the milk carton to the appropriate height of the taper candle. Fill with crushed ice.

3. Add Peppermint essential oil to ice.

4. Sprinkle glitter into the cooling paraffin and stir.

5. Pour paraffin into the carton and let cool.

6. After it has cooled, pour off the water and tear away the carton to reveal your sparkling new creation.

Index

CPSIA information can be obtained
at www.ICGtesting.com
Printed in the USA
BVOW09s1655210218
508745BV00005B/317/P